P9-EMF-974

A Manual for Culturally-adapted Social Marketing

A Manual for Culturally-adapted Social Marketing

Health and Population

Edited by

T. Scarlett Epstein

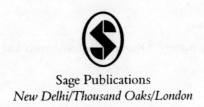

Sage Publications
New Delhi/Thousand Oaks/London

Copyright © T. Scarlett Epstein, 1999

All rights reserved. No part of this book may be reproduced or utilised in any form or by any means, electronic or mechanical, including photocopying, recording or by any information storage or retrieval system, without permission in writing from the publisher.

First published in 1999 by

Sage Publications India Pvt Ltd
M-32 Market, Greater Kailash Part - I
New Delhi-110 048

Sage Publications Inc.
2455 Teller Road
Thousand Oaks, California 91320

Sage Publications Ltd
6 Bonhill Street
London EC2A 4PU

Published by Tejeshwar Singh for Sage Publications India Pvt Ltd, typeset by Siva Math Setters, Chennai and printed at Chaman Enterprises, Delhi.

Library of Congress Cataloging-in-Publication Data

A manual for culturally-adapted social marketing: health and population/edited by T. Scarlett Epstein.
     p. cm. (p)
    Includes bibliographical references.

    1. Social marketing. I. Epstein, T. Scarlett (Trude Scarlett)
  HF5414.M38   658.8—dc21   1999   99–23261

ISBN: 0–7619–9334–7 (US-PB)
      81–7036–799–9 (India-PB)

Sage Production Team: Abantika Chatterji, Dharam Chand Sharma and Santosh Rawat

This manual is dedicated to all those who devote their energies
to encourage behavioural changes that are undoubtedly
in the people's own best interest

Contents

PART I: INTRODUCTION

PART II: CULTURALLY-ADAPTED SOCIAL MARKETING (CASM) IN THEORY AND PRACTICE

PART III: SOME CASM CASE STUDIES

E.   A UK Drugs Information Study Focusing on Children Aged 9–10   *Hermione Lovel*

PART IV: A CASM EXPERIMENTAL EXERCISE

List of Tables

List of Figures

List of Charts

Acknowledgements

I owe a great debt to the Health and Population Division of the UK Department for International Development and the Commonwealth Secretariat for supporting the production of this manual. I also appreciate very much the collaborative spirit shown by all the contributors to this publication, who patiently responded to the many questions I raised on their papers and never complained about my continued demands for further improvements and more revisions. My special thanks go out to Professor E. L. Roberto who, as one of the world's pioneers in social marketing, kindly agreed in spite of all his many commitments to vet the first drafts of chapters 2, 5 and 6 and let us have his critical comments, in the light of which Professor Jha (their author) revised his contribution. I wish to express my gratitude also to all those other individuals, who in one way or the other, helped in the task of compiling and editing this publication. There are far too many of them to name each individually: I only hope that the finished product will make them feel that their efforts have been worthwhile.

This manual represents a necessary sequel to the *Manual for Culturally-Adapted Market Research in the Development Process* (Epstein 1988) which showed **why** developers should treat their target audiences in the same way as businesses treat their potential clients and the *Training Manual for Development Market Research Investigators* (Epstein, et al. 1991), which outlined **how** such research needs to be conducted. Because the findings of this type of market research indicated that people often behave in ways harmful to themselves, particularly concerning their own health, it seemed imperative to provide succinct guidelines about **how** to conduct culturally-adapted social marketing (CASM). Commercial **marketing** had already shown that it could successfully influence behaviour, therefore, such marketing strategies began to be adopted into a social and non-market setting over 30 years ago. But until recently social marketing has been used mainly in Western industrial societies—mostly in the United States—where there now exist considerable numbers of such specialised agencies. In many developing countries, where socially desirable behavioural changes are desperately needed, social marketing experts and the funds to pay for them are regrettably still extremely scarce. Many well-intentioned organisations and individuals working in the Third World are trying their best to effect behavioural changes that are in the best interest of their target audiences, but they often lack the knowledge of how to do so in a culturally-appropriate manner and/or the funds to recruit experts to help them.

This manual, by providing guidelines for the conduct of CASM as well as detailed case materials of projects that applied CASM in different Third World societies as part of their attempts to improve mother and child health in particular and reproductive health in general should, therefore, enable development practitioners to make enlightened judgements about the pros and cons of CASM and to decide for themselves whether and how they may use it in their attempts to improve not only levels of health but the quality of life in particular among the poorest people. Whether the manual will in fact succeed in helping development practitioners in achieving these laudable objectives remains to be seen.

T. Scarlett Epstein

Part I

Introduction

Chapter 1

About this Manual

T. Scarlett Epstein

1.1 WHAT IS THE PURPOSE OF THIS MANUAL?

This manual aims to help different types of project field staff—particularly those working in the context of mother and child issues and reproductive health—to succeed in their tasks. Many such field staff in different parts of the world often bitterly complain that the people who they are trying to help refuse to undergo the necessary behavioural changes involved. As a qualified development economist and anthropologist who has spent years personally conducting and/or directing socio-economic micro-societal studies in Third World countries, I tried to find out why so many development projects fail to reach their objectives—though of course this is not meant to imply that there are not also many projects that succeed. But the fact remains that a large proportion fail, which means that a lot of still badly-needed resources are wasted.

I soon discovered that projects that were not in tune with their target audiences' aspirations had a tendency to collapse after the initial external and often expatriate input was withdrawn. Well-meaning experts usually decide what project should be put where and it is implemented without anyone ever trying to put the proposition to the people who will be affected, to sound out their views on it. Project designers may be experts in technical aspects but they only rarely know the mind-set of their target people or the socio-cultural setting into which their projects have to fit. Examples abound that illustrate the importance of this point. Many projects have thus come to represent alien grafts which affected societies sooner or later reject. Hence the wastage of development resources.

1.2 CLIENT-LED RATHER THAN TOP-DOWN DEVELOPMENT

The disenchantment with this top-down development strategy led to the emphasis on 'participatory development', to involve target audiences in the developmental decision-making process so that the help they get is in line with their own sets of priorities. A variety of different types of 'participatory research and development' methods have become established in different field situations.

My own contribution in this context has been to examine how businesses succeed in **selling** their products, while the same people who make those purchases often reject what developers offer them **free of charge**. It soon became obvious that businesses that succeed do so because in their marketing they adopt the consumer's perspective—their marketing is client-led. To get to know their customers' mind-set, businesses have learnt that they must base their marketing strategies on sound market research. This fact suggests that for development projects to succeed they also need to be client-led; in other words, developers should treat their target audiences—even if they do not pay for what they are getting—in the same way and with the same respect as businesses treat their potential clients.

1.2.1   Culturally-adapted Social Market Research (CASOMAR)

To spread this gospel I published two manuals: the first in 1988 in which I targeted developers, trying to make them realise **WHY** they should use social market research and adopt client-led practices, and the second in 1991, which sets out **HOW** to conduct culturally-adapted social market research (CASOMAR).

However, from some of the CASOMAR findings it soon became obvious that people's behaviour and their aspirations are often not in their own best interest: they smoke and get lung cancer; they are promiscuous and contract AIDS, they practise environmental degradation and thereby jeopardise their own future and that of their descendants. It is this self-destructive tendency in people which seems to frustrate many well-intentioned developers and results in project failures. Thus, there is an urgent need to find ways and means to get people to begin to behave along lines that are in their own best interest.

1.3   HOW CAN SOCIALLY DESIRABLE BEHAVIOURAL CHANGES BE ENCOURAGED?

Many solutions have been proposed for the numerous social problems which world societies face and, typically, there are disagreements on how best to solve problems as diverse as illiteracy, drug abuse, high maternal mortality and environmental degradation. Often calls are made for the launch of educational campaigns to change public attitudes and behaviour.

1.3.1   Education

Many perceive education as the panacea for all social ills. Education is certainly a useful means to bring about desirable social change (e.g., the emancipation of women) but it is rarely effective in the short-term. The content of education is also often not appropriate to lead to the desired social changes. Moreover, a large proportion of the poorest people want education for their children not for the benefit to be derived from better knowledge and understanding, but because they consider it as a passport to employment. Education for education's or welfare's sake appears to be a luxury only wealthier societies can and do afford. In many parts of the world, there exists a correlation between the socio-economic standing of a household and the formal educational levels of its children, and women usually have lower educational achievements than men.

1.3.2 Social Marketing

Thus education has not proved to be very effective in achieving desirable social objectives at least within one lifetime. By contrast, commercial marketing has scored many successes in securing behavioural changes within short periods of time.

The idea that commercial sector marketing may be successfully applied in a wider socio-political setting was first mooted in the late 1960s, when marketing experts realised that the basic goal of marketing is to influence behaviour, whether that behaviour is buying a pair of jeans, voting for a specific policy or a politician, discontinuing smoking or using drugs. Politicians have been quick to realise the advantages the adoption of marketing strategies offer if they base their publicity campaigns on carefully conducted opinion polls. The successes scored by adopting marketing strategies into a non-market setting encouraged the richer developed societies to devote large budgets to the marketing of socially desirable causes, for instance, the reduction of smoking, HIV/AIDS and the promotion of cancer smear tests for women.

In the poorer developing nations the state allocates hardly any money to bring about behavioural changes by means of social marketing campaigns. This is reflected, for instance, in their continuous high rate of smoking, comparatively low average expectation of life and high mortality rates, particularly infant mortality.

Developers have only more recently begun to appreciate the positive role market research and marketing strategies can play in the implementation process of their projects. As target segmentation—which divides target societies into culturally-homogenous groups (see Figure 2.1)—forms a major part of marketing activities, it becomes necessary to establish cost- and time-effective methods to ensure that market research and marketing is culturally-appropriate. This has led to the cultural adaptation of social market research (CASOMAR) and social marketing (CASM) by using **project-specific key cultural variables** (see 4.2.1) in compiling cultural profiles of different target societies and their segments.

1.3.3 CASM and Participatory Research

CASM is one of a number of participatory research and development approaches as it uses culturally-adapted social market research (CASOMAR) to elicit the target society's own project-related expectations and aspirations; it differs from most other 'participatory development' methods only in as much as it does not recommend discarding or changing the project to meet client expectations whenever CASOMAR findings indicate a difference between people's aspirations and what experts consider on undisputable evidence to be the best for the target audience. In case of such divergence, CASOMAR suggests the use of social marketing in collaboration with the local people to ensure behavioural changes that are in their own best interest.

Developers working with government and non-government or voluntary organisations (NGOs or VOs) often encounter the problem of wanting to introduce socially desirable behavioural changes among their target societies, without having much of an idea of how to do this. Only a few of them know about the advantages social marketing offers in this context or what it involves. They also do not have the funds to employ relevant experts to help them achieve their project objectives.

This manual attempts to provide advice and guidelines to all those concerned with grassroots level development on how best to encourage socially desirable behavioural changes among their target audiences. It is important here to stress that CASM can help not only in working with villagers or urban dwellers but also in dealing with government departments or corporations. Using CASM can help to change behaviour at all levels of society.

The overriding purpose of this CASM manual is to enable developers to find out what CASM is all about so that they can decide whether, where and how they can apply it to help ensure that their laudable work will reach its socially desirable objectives.

1.4   A USER-FRIENDLY MANUAL

This is a manual with a difference—it aims to be user-friendly by having the following features:

Contributors: *The team of contributors is composed of an unusual mixture of developmentally-oriented academicians and experienced development practitioners.*

Easy-to read style: *Contributions are written in easily understood colloquial English and jargon has been avoided as far as possible.*

Translations: *It is hoped that before long this manual will be translated into different vernaculars to help developers who are not fluent in English.*

Graphics: *To illustrate certain phenomena with drawings, Ray Evans was recruited; he is an artist working with the Unit of Art in Medicine at the University of Manchester, England.*

Recommended reading: *Instead of including quotations and references, which often make reading tedious—lists of recommended reading appear at the end of most contributions for those who thirst for more, relevant information.*

Pilot testing: *Some chapters have been pilot tested in India and the Philippines and revised accordingly. As it was a lengthy process to compile the various contributions to this manual and to avoid further delay of publication, no full pilot test has been conducted.*

Questionnaire: *A brief questionnaire is included and it will be greatly appreciated if readers complete and return it to the publishers. The information gained from the completed questionnaires will help not only to further improve future editions of the manual and ensure that it becomes truly client-led, but it will also provide the basis for establishing a network among development practitioners interested in CASM. This may then lead to the publication of a CASM newsletter.*

Bio-data: *Summary bio-data of each of the contributors are given to put readers in a better position to evaluate each paper and detect possible biases.*

1.5   WHAT DOES THIS MANUAL CONTAIN?

It consists of four Parts and an Appendix:

1.5.1   Part I: Introduction

1.5.2   Part II: Culturally-adapted Social Marketing in Theory and Practice

This includes five chapters contributed by two academicians setting out **WHY** and **HOW** CASM should be conducted.

Chapters 2, 5 and 6 which examine the different features of social marketing are contributed by Dr M. Jha, Professor of Marketing at the Indian·Institute of Management at Bangalore. By using the example of

Sanjeevani, an NGO that aims to recruit blood donors, he describes in detail what is involved in the conduct of CASM.

Chapter 3 sets out the participatory nature of social market research as an integral part of social marketing and Chapter 4 discusses the importance of cultural sensitivity in any marketing venture and recounts the methods by which this can be ensured.

These five chapters outline the norms of CASOMAR and CASM. Realising that practice often deviates from the norm, development practitioners were asked to share their experience in their use of CASM as part of projects focusing on mother and child issues and reproductive health. The six case studies refer to projects conducted in Africa, Asia, Latin America and the Pacific. None of them show that they followed step-by-step the CASOMAR and CASM course of action set out in Chapters 2 to 6; lack of acquaintance with these procedures and/or practical necessities made these practitioners use some and adapt other parts of textbook CASM. This widens the spectrum of CASM activities and should help readers choose the course of action they consider best to pursue.

1.5.3 Part III: Some CASM Case Material

This is made up of six CASM case studies, the authors of each of which were directly involved in the projects they relate.

1.5.3.1 *A Mother-child Health Project*

This is discussed by Marie-Therese Feuerstein (see Case Study A), who acted as consultant to a 'Safe Motherhood' project—part of a government integrated rural development programme among the Simbu in the Highlands of Papua New Guinea. This 'Safe Motherhood' project began by collecting background data on the Simbu culture and other relevant available materials. Through different channels and by varying means the project effectively elicited what different sections of the target society thought about the child-bearing experience in particular and family planning in general. It emerged that many Simbu men were ignorant about these topics (see A.7.6 and A.7.7). Initial enquiries led to target segmentation and a focus on village health workers on the one hand and young married couples on the other. By imaginative cultural-adaptation of the content and means of communication to the different target segments (see A.9) the project ensured community and health workers' commitment and succeeded in encouraging the practice of safe motherhood. However, it faced serious problems with the higher levels of the government health administration, which proved extremely difficult to solve (see A.11), and about which the project team could do little but accept it as a 'given constraint' to its success (A.5).

1.5.3.2 *Three Reproductive Health Projects*

- Ajit Mani and Susan Thomas (see Case Study B) recount a 'Family Planning Project' in a S. Indian village, where after initial inquiries the family planning team used social marketing to overcome or at least reduce the impact of many of the cultural factors that adversely affected the population's reproductive health. A SWOT analysis pointed out the strengths, weaknesses, opportunities and threats with which the project had to grapple. An effective marketing-mix was designed by practising careful target segmentation—i.e., boys clubs, girls clubs, women's groups, educated unemployed—to divide the village population into socially recognisable and meaningful groups.

Different types of promotion activities were used to remove the taboo from discussing sex and reproduction: village meetings chaired and addressed by respected female officials, family planning posters displayed at strategic points, condoms advertised in local petty shops and film shows on reproduction organised.

Having found that the older village men represented their toughest opponents and knowing that these men longed for entertainment, the project arranged the performance of a culturally-appropriate drama in which the Gods answered the prayers of a woman to be spared more pregnancies and decreed that the husband would bear the children. The men had to watch a man going through a painful delivery to bear an ugly demon. This was a traumatic experience for these men and radically changed their attitudes towards fertility and the relationship with their wives. It is interesting to note here that a similar approach was successfully used in the PNG 'Safe Motherhood Project' when two men did a role play of a pregnant woman in labour and childbirth (see A.9.5.9) which made men realise that they should know far more than they did about childbirth. Indices used to evaluate the Bilekahalli project appear to indicate its success: the proportion of family planning acceptors increased considerably and infant mortality and the average size of family reduced. But without valid comparative data right from the outset of the project from villages that had not been subjected to such project activities it was impossible to say how much of the changes were due to the project and how much to other influences.

- Patricio Mora (see Case Study C) outlines a joint PLAN INTERNATIONAL/UNFPA 'Mother-Child Health' project which he directs in the mountains of southern Ecuador; it was still on-going when he wrote his paper. His familiarity with CASM is illustrated by the systematic way this project has been organised: Objectives were clearly defined; a baseline survey including qualitative and quantitative inquiries was conducted jointly by project staff, official health workers and local villagers. This was followed by a culturally-adapted feedback to the communities (see C.2.2), the selection and training of local voluntary health providers (VHP) and the formation of women's groups. To ensure project sustainability a lot of attention was paid to encouraging socially desirable behavioural changes not only among the targeted village people but also among all the other relevant individuals and institutions, such as the local Catholic priest and the Ministry of Health, to establish a community health system. The project, for instance, encouraged changes in the Organisational Structure of the Ministry of Health (see C.5) by setting up a working partnership with the health department establishment. This harmonious relationship is apparently due to the project staff treating their official partners as if they were the final consumers; their expectations such as staff training and computerisation of health data were examined and arrangements were made accordingly. It is in this particular aspect that this project differs from most others of its kind, the staff of which still naively assume that health department officials must willy-nilly act altruistically in the interest of the project and get frustrated if this does not occur. The Ecuador project avoided this mistake and looked upon the relevant health officials as another target segment and began by examining their expectations and then tried to meet their aspirations, for instance, by providing a manual and training for Ministry of Health staff (see C.6.1). During the brief period of its existence, the project managed by using the 'appropriate market mix' to lay a sound foundation for its ultimate success which, however, will become apparent only in future years.

- A Community Self-Help Programme in Kenya (see Case Study D) which used CASM to reduce the incidence and suffering from HIV/AIDS/STD is presented here by Marie-Therese Feuerstein and Anne Owiti. The increasing number of AIDS orphans was the main stimulus to the programme. Anne Owiti, a nurse-midwife had encountered many cases of AIDS/STD victims who desperately needed home-based care and support. The programme began by identifying and exploring a few key cultural variables (KCVs) such as sexuality norms, secrecy surrounding HIV/AIDS and confidentiality, and compiling a cultural profile of the selected slum dweller target. A carefully conducted CASOMAR highlighted the problems caused by high levels of unemployment and extreme poverty and deprivation. On the basis of the finding the selected slum dwellers were divided into different socially meaningful segments and different strategies designed to reach the different target segments—for instance home-based care (see D.5.1) and action to help AIDS orphans (see D.5.2). This has led to a widespread acceptance of the use of condoms, which were distributed free. Like so many other Third World development projects this one too encountered many constraints (see D.7), particularly of a financial nature. Feuerstein and Owiti widen the field of their focus and provide a fascinating discussion of how the incidence of HIV/AIDS may be reduced among floating populations such as migrant workers and refugees and out-of-school and socially apart youth. They give examples of on-going CASM activities in different parts of the world. In Chile, a board game 'Learning about AIDS' has become an important learning device (see Chart D.2). More such imaginative CASM is urgently needed to reduce the spread of AIDS.

1.5.3.3   A UK Drugs Information Project

Hermione Lovel (see Case Study E) presents a UK Drugs Information Study focusing on children aged 9–10. The study directors started with the assumption that social marketing offers the most effective approach to inform young children about the problems arising from drug intake because it begins by trying to learn all about the mind-set of the target group. They divided the group into different socially identifiable segments: school children aged 9–10 were the primary target and parents and teachers made up the secondary target. In-depth CASOMAR was conducted of these different target segments in three stages: The listening stage, the interpretation stage and the piloting stage (see E.2). Different techniques were used to elicit information from the different target segments: children, the primary target, were asked to participate in 'draw and write' techniques (E.3.1.1) and the self-portrait exercises (see E.3.1.2), whereas parents and teachers, the secondary target, were subjected to in-depth interviews which were conducted according to a predesigned discussion-guide (see E.3.2). The findings of Stage one highlighted the advantages that will accrue from getting children to construct a small 'Me Box' (see E.3) as part of their schooling. Nearly every child personalised his/her book and showed creativity and self-esteem in its production. The exercise was found enjoyable by students and teachers alike and the analysis of the content proved very illuminating. The resulting booklets were pilot tested with parents and teachers, who all agreed that they were interesting and useful. This truly client-led project throws into relief the advantages to be derived from a culturally-appropriate social marketing approach in the compilation of effective drugs information materials.

1.5.3.4   AIDPLUS (INDIA) Raises Funds Project

Ajit Mani and Susan Thomas (see Case Study F) were involved in a fund-raising project when the Indian subsidiary of a large British NGO—to which they give the pseudonym AIDPLUS—aimed to raise substantial funds within India. The CASOMAR with which the project started indicated significant differences in the cultural assumptions of charity that prevail in Western societies on the one hand and among Hindus on the other (see F.2.1.1 and F.2.1.2); it also yielded information on 'donating behaviour motivation' (see F.2.3).

All this made AIDPLUS broaden their objectives from concentrating solely on fund-raising to creating interest and involvement in India in the work of AIDPLUS. AIDPLUS (INDIA) established a publicity department headed by a young woman with experience of work with an advertising agency who was helped by two British consultants (see F.4). They decided to concentrate on the production and sale of greetings cards (see F.4.1) and on a direct mail appeal (see F.4.2). The results of the marketing campaign (see F.5) proved that the greetings cards was a failure and the direct mail appeal a great success. It emerged that many young, upwardly mobile professionals quickly became dedicated supporters because it gave them a feeling of being able to influence, at least to some extent, the chaotic conditions prevailing around them. As most NGOs based in the Third World continuously face financial problems, this case study should be of interest to many individuals engaged in voluntary activities.

1.5.4 Part IV: A CASM Experimental Exercise

This exercise has three objectives:

- To offer readers an incentive to engage in CASM
- To encourage readers to try their hand at designing a CASM strategy
- To tap the brains and experience of a wide audience to find a CASM strategy that will effectively reduce the harmful practice of female genital mutilation

The value and success of this CASM manual depends on how much interest it will arouse and how useful readers find it. Please therefore:

Complete and return the enclosed questionnaire with your critical comments **and** *pose any further questions you may have regarding CASM*

1.6 RECOMMENDED READING

Andreasen, A.R. (1994). 'Social Marketing: Definition and Domain', *Journal of Marketing and Public Policy*, Spring, pp. 108–14.

Andreasen, A.R. (1995). *Marketing Social Change*, Jossey-Bass, San Francisco.

Fine, S. (ed.) (1990). *Social Marketing: Promoting the causes of public and nonprofit agencies*, Allyn and Bacon, Boston.

Kotler, P. and **A.R. Andreasen** (1996). *Strategic Marketing for Nonprofit Organizations*, Prentice Hall, Englewood Cliffs, NJ.

Kotler, P. and **E. Roberto** (1989). *Social Marketing: Strategies for Changing Public Behaviour*, The Free Press, New York.

Rothchild, M.D. (1979). 'Marketing Communications in Non-business situations or Why It's So Hard to Sell Brotherhood like Soap', *Journal of Marketing*, Spring, pp. 11–20.

Schwartz, B. (1994, May). 'Social Marketing for Gender Equity in Bangladesh', *Social Marketing Quarterly*, I, 3.

Part II

Culturally-adapted Social Marketing (CASM) in Theory and Practice

Chapter 2

What is Culturally-adapted
Social Marketing (CASM)?

Mithileshwar Jha

> *'Why can't you sell brotherhood like you sell soaps?'*
> *(Wiebe, 1951–52)*

An Indian non-government organisation (NGO), working for slum and street children, used these children's inborn artistic talents to produce greetings cards with paintings done by them. The profile of the child artist was mentioned at the back of these nicely printed cards. After facing some problems in selling these cards through book and gift shops, it involved multiple channels, including student volunteers, to sell thousands of cards generating substantial resources for the organisation.

A cancer screening programme developed innovative incentives (non-monetary) for its participants—volunteer physicians—so that its target clients, mostly poor and dispersed all over the city, could have easy access to a cancer screening facility. They also placed advertisements in local newspapers, and used the help of physicians and opinion leaders in various organisations (particularly union leaders in various industrial units) to create awareness among the target clients (persons above 40 years of age) about the desirability of cancer screening. The advertisements featured cured cancer patients with the message 'life after cancer is worth living'. It also said 'cancer, if detected early, is curable'. The organisation decided to provide full confidentiality to patients. It also decided to charge scaled fees for the services provided: very nominal charges for the poor and slightly higher fees for others.

These are just a few examples of the use of commercial marketing and management practices for the benefit of individuals, groups and society. These are systematic attempts at bringing about social change. These are situations involving social marketing.

Kotler and Roberto, the pioneers in social marketing (1989) define it as:

> *...A social change management technology involving the design, implementation and control of programmes aimed at increasing the acceptability of a social idea or practice in one or more groups of target adopters. It utilises the concepts of market segmentation, consumer research, product concept development and testing, direct communication, facilitation, incentives and exchange theory to maximise the target adopters response. (p. 24)*

Social marketing focuses on enhancing the acceptability of socially relevant ideas and practices for social change. It requires appreciation of the following:

- It deals with enhancing the acceptability of a socially desirable idea/practice (such as family planning, anti-smoking campaign, spreading AIDS awareness and prevention techniques and blood donation).

■ It focuses on specific target publics (e.g., donors, target users, motivators and facilitators, each of whom may be treated as a separate constituency and reached through specialised channels and efforts).

■ It requires understanding the needs, wants and demands of the target audience, their motivations and aspirations, their relationships, and decision-making processes and roles.

■ It requires systematic understanding of the above through culturally-adapted market research.

■ It requires grouping together (segmenting) target audiences with similar response characteristics.

■ It requires developing a total offer consisting of product (such as goods, services and ideas), communication, pricing/value, proposition/incentives (both tangible and intangible), facilitation through logistics and other ways.

■ Finally, it requires continuous monitoring and upgrading of the offer to ensure participant satisfaction and the desired response.

2.1 DIFFERENCES BETWEEN COMMERCIAL MARKETING AND CULTURALLY-ADAPTED SOCIAL MARKETING

CASM activities have several peculiarities compared to conventional commercial marketing activities. Some of these are:

■ Commercial marketers target the client segment which is most willing to accept their offer. CASM marketers have to deal with negative demand in many situations. In many cases the individual may not even perceive a direct benefit, for example, environmental issues, family planning and health measures.

■ Customers normally pay for the goods and services in commercial marketing. Clients and donors in CASM (who partly or fully pay for the services offered) may be completely different entities with different needs and motivations.

■ In commercial marketing, particularly in large organisations, a complex organisational structure deals with seemingly simple issues. In CASM, complex issues are usually dealt with by very simplistic structures.

■ The resources available to CASM managers are generally much smaller compared to the magnitude of the task involved.

■ The nature of behavioural changes over time for CASM marketers is more drastic compared to everyday commercial marketing.

■ Pleasing end-customers may not necessarily coincide with meeting donor expectation; despite being successful in achieving client objectives, the organisation may not be viable.

■ The task in CASM is not to create dependence. So, instead of retaining clients, the focus may be to empower clients to be self-reliant and for the organisation to move on to other segments or tasks.

2.2 WHAT DEVELOPMENT MANAGERS CAN LEARN FROM COMMERCIAL MARKETING

Development managers can plan and implement their activities better by learning from commercial marketing while planning and implementing CASM. CASM, like commercial marketing, begins with relevant research, the findings of which provide the basis for the subsequent marketing plan as set out below:

■ Situation analyses involve SWOT (strength, weakness, opportunity and threat) analysis, and competence analyses: these help to identify key opportunities and issues.

■ Setting objectives both short- and long-term (based on the above analyses), qualitative and quantitative, which provide standards for performance.

■ Developing a CASM strategy and mix, which involves deciding on the choice of target segments of clients, choice of image, relationship with different target segments, the broad approach to reach and influence the target segments, and deciding on the 8P's of the CASM-mix (namely, product, place, price, promotion, people, process, politics and pace).

8P's

The example of an NGO-operated blood bank, which we name 'Sanjeevani' (to keep its anonymity), is used here to illustrate how to develop a CASM strategy.

2.2.1 Situation Analyses

After having conducted and processed the relevant CASOMAR data (see Chapters 3 and 4) the next step is to prepare a SWOT analysis. This is illustrated in Table 2.1 with reference to Sanjeevani.

Table 2.1
SWOT for Sanjeevani

Strengths	*Weaknesses*
★ Committed founders	★ Poor resources
★ Small, qualified staff	★ High staff turnover
★ Good local reputation	★ Lack of organisation skills
	★ Poor public relations
Opportunities	*Threats*
★ Local institutions with positive outlook towards blood donations	★ Fear of AIDS
★ Fear of AIDS, etc., forcing potential donors to search for credible blood banks	★ Youth wings of political parties organising blood donation camps in the area with lots of publicity but little concern, resulting in apprehensions in the public mind
★ Poor reputation of government and other local blood banks	★ Public apathy
	★ Other charitable activities

Considering its strengths and weaknesses and looking at the opportunities offered by the client groups and the threats coming from the environment including other competing organisations, Sanjeevani's management came to the following conclusion:

● Being small, with limited resources and a good local reputation, its basic competence was in targeting local institutions (schools, colleges and corporate offices in the area).

● With limited resources, it was possible for the founders to build good personalised relationships with the few high potential institutions.

- They estimated that these institutions, numbering about fifty, had a potential blood donor population of about 5,000 individuals. If about 20 per cent of these could be tapped on a quarterly basis, it could yield 1,000 bottles/pouches of 250 ml blood each. With greater effort this could be improved further.
- Sanjeevani also decided to overcome its weaknesses on the personnel front by enlisting the support of some reputed local physicians and final year medical students of a local medical college (only a small, dedicated band).
- It tried to convert threats into opportunities by enlisting the support of local youth clubs and other charitable organisations, which provided good infrastructural and publicity support (in business terms these may be called strategic alliances).

2.2.2   Setting Objectives

Sanjeevani's management set the following short-term and long-term objectives for itself:

a) Short-term objectives (1–2 years)
  - To collect and distribute about 500 litres of blood during the next year.
  - To create community awareness about the need for blood donation in about 50 per cent of the target clients (about 2,500 individuals).
  - To educate those aware, about the misconceptions surrounding blood donation.
  - To create an image of Sanjeevani as the safest and most preferred organisation to donate blood to.
  - To create an image of Sanjeevani among potential volunteers, institutions and other facilitators as a preferred organisation with which to work.

b) Long-term objectives (3–5 years)
  - To develop into a leading blood bank with an annual collection and distribution of 5,000 litres of blood, through a chain of affiliated centres.
  - To develop into a diagnostic centre offering advanced diagnostic facilities, at nominal costs, with the poor as the preferred clientele.
  - To attract and retain professionally competent and service-oriented personnel at all levels.
  - To establish and sustain Sanjeevani as a dependable, safe, service-oriented friend for the interacting public and its own personnel.

2.2.3   CASM Strategy for Sanjeevani

It consisted of decisions of the viable image Sanjeevani wanted to project and the broad approach to achieve the desired image.

Client Segments

Keeping in mind its competence and opportunities, Sanjeevani's management considered the following client segments (see Figure 2.1):

Figure 2.1
Sanjeevani Client Segments

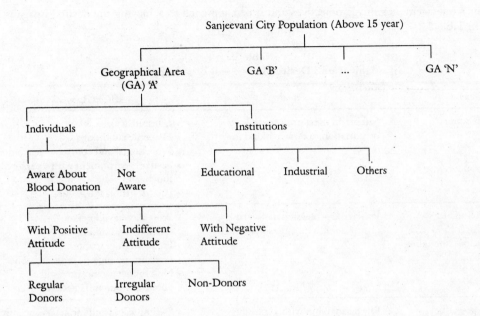

After long discussions among Sanjeevani's staff, it was decided that the focus should initially be on educational and large and medium industrial units (in terms of number of employees) in the geographical areas 'A' and 'B'. This was done keeping in mind the following:

* Short-term objectives.
* Limited resources resulting in limited quality access.
* Importance of awareness, education and building positive relationships based on trust and positive experience.
* Need to develop institutional members into community volunteers in the long run.
* To keep the logistics and cost of operations within its limits without compromising on the quality of service.

In the long run, Sanjeevani had plans of expanding to cover all individuals in the areas 'A' and 'B' and gradually the whole city. It had plans to expand its premises into a full-fledged diagnostic centre and start operations in other areas in alliance with other NGOs.

It identified a mix of clients. They were:

* Target blood donors (identified in Figure 2.1).
* Initiators, influencers (such as heads of the institutions, union leaders and student leaders).
* Facilitators (youth leaders, leading doctors, school teachers, personnel in associate charitable organisations).

★ Its own personnel, whose motivation, service quality and commitment to the cause were essential for a recurring positive client experience.

2.2.3.1 Image and Broad Approach vis-à-vis Different Client Groups

Sanjeevani's management's image objectives and broad approach to achieving the desired image is summarised in Table 2.2.

Table 2.2
Sanjeevani's Desired Image and Broad Approach

Target Group	Image	Broad Approach
1. Blood donors	Safest and most preferred organisation to donate blood to	★ Latest instruments ★ Hygienic conditions ★ Professional and courteous personnel ★ Festive environment with a personal touch, and ★ Post-donation follow-up
2. and 3. Initiators, influencers and facilitators (including regulators)	Preferred, professional charitable organisation with a personal touch	★ Professional and personal relationship building ★ Frequent interaction ★ Praising and giving credit in public ★ Non monetary incentives like public honour and citation
4. Own personnel	Fair partnership with a socially desirable objective	★ Decent wages and monetary incentive ★ Modern gadgets and training to use them ★ Professional pride ★ Freedom, and ★ Ownership feeling

2.3 CASM-MIX FOR SANJEEVANI

CASM-mix deals with specific actionable elements of the programme used by social marketers. These elements are classified here as the 8Ps of CASM, namely, Product, Place, Price, Promotion, People, Process, Politics and Pace.

These, as used by Sanjeevani, are being highlighted below: (For the sake of simplicity it is being done for only the blood donor group.)

(A) Product: Sanjeevani defined its product characteristics in the following manner:

★ It had to convince the potential donors of the desirability of the **idea of** blood donation. This may require changing/reinforcing existing beliefs, attitudes and values.

★ It had to persuade potential donors with positive attitudes to **act**, i.e., to donate blood, and motivate others to donate.

* It had to make potential donors come to one or another of its venues (premises, mobile vans or camps) to donate blood.
* It had to give donors certificates and possibly some tangible evidence to show that the blood donated would be used for a meaningful cause together with a letter of thanks, to reinforce the act by providing a tangible evidence of the noble act.

Sanjeevani's management realised that they were not dealing with just 'blood donation' as a product, but were dealing with the idea of 'giving', 'community and citizenship values' along with the tangible 'blood donation'.

They also appreciated the fact that the first phone call, personal interactions, facilities at the base office and camp site, the appearance and conduct of professionals during the donation process, the commendation certificate, the post-donation letter and subsequent oral and written requests—everything contributed towards this intangible and tangible product. Target blood donors judged quality of the final product on the basis of each of these interactions.

(B) Place: This refers to logistics and all the activities to provide access to the target donors. Sanjeevani decided on the following in this regard:

* It would locate donation camps at an easily accessible public institution or at the target donors' office premises.
* It would use a mobile van, with the facility to receive blood from two donors simultaneously, for smaller organisations.
* It decided to carry folding cots, partitions, mattresses, clean white bed sheets and other accessories in the same van.
* It decided to motivate facilitators to offer snacks and beverages to the donors at the site, (being culturally sensitive, it decided to offer hot beverages, a preferred option after blood donation as per local belief).
* It decided to use trained volunteers and competent, courteous medical staff to attend to blood donors.
* It decided to use clean, disinfected, spacious, airy halls for the purpose.
* Separate counters were to be opened for registration, blood testing, blood donation, snacks and for issuing commendation certificates.
* Counsellors were also to be made available to answer any queries/doubts.
* Finally, separate areas to rest in were to be made available for those who felt giddy.

The guiding principle in place-related decisions was easy access, clean, hygienic and friendly environment, personal touch and cost-effectiveness while maintaining high quality service standards.

(C) Price: Sanjeevani knew that although donors were not charged any fee, they were paying hidden prices, like cost of their time, cost of transport to the camp, psychological risk of contamination, including the fear of AIDS, and fear of post-donation weakness. It decided to offer guaranteed safety, used the best possible accessories, disposed of used syringes in the presence of the donors and hired credible professionals to be seen to offer quality service. One reason for Sanjeevani focusing its attention on a limited client segment was its concern and commitment to offer its donors service of the highest value.

It also made sure that its personnel were paid decent wages and honorarium and were treated with utmost professional respect. It used its professional network to provide visibility and career advancement to its personnel. It acknowledged committed performance by publicly honouring its personnel.

(D) Promotion: (such as publicity, public relations and advertising): Sanjeevani, having a relatively small, focused clientele, believed more in personal communication. However, it effectively used the following means to create awareness, persuade target donors and sustain their interest:

* Placing small, awareness creating advertisements in local newspapers, in space donated by charitable organisations and individuals.
* Organising lectures at institutions and local clubs, educating people and clearing doubts/misapprehensions.
* Distributing leaflets and putting up posters informing people of the date, time and venue of blood donation camps.
* Using volunteers to mobilise and bring donors to the camp site.
* Involving local physicians, convincing potential donors and informing and activating them.
* Involving freelance creative persons in designing advertisements, posters, letters, commendation certificates, and so on.
* Involving social workers, teachers, nurses/midwives, volunteer students and its own personnel in eliciting pre- and post-donation feelings.
* Using street theatre to convey the message of blood donation and to remove apprehension.

(E) People: This refers to the organisation's personnel. Sanjeevani's management appreciated the basic fact that you cannot satisfy your donor clients and other facilitators unless you have **competent, courteous and committed** personnel. Their recruitment, training, development and motivation processes focused on attracting and retaining a small band of committed personnel. There was a high turnover of volunteers and other part-time personnel, but each one ensured that they trained sufficient replacements.

(F) Process: Sanjeevani had taken help from volunteer management professionals to develop simple and effective processes. Some of these were:

* A one-page simple registration form, which had relevant details about the donor. This could be completed in 5–8 minutes.
* It had computerised its data base and had the names, addresses and other relevant details of about 2,000 individuals and 30 institutions. This data base was updated every six months. Efforts continued to further expand the list.
* Sanjeevani had developed a separate data base for professionals, volunteers, facilitators, and others.
* It had simple handbooks which were used for volunteer training. They contained relevant information on important queries regarding blood donation in a questionnaire form and checklists suggesting do's and don'ts.
* On joining, volunteers were given a half-day orientation programme. They first worked as understudies to experienced volunteers before being given independent assignments.
* At the blood donation camp site, the layout for various activities like reception and registration counter, blood testing counter, blood donation section, rest area, snacks distribution counter, and commendation certificate counter were carefully planned and organised.

Volunteers greeted potential blood donors on arrival, helped them complete the form, guided them through various sections with utmost attention and care, without being intrusive.

* One of the senior founder partners of Sanjeevani always made it a point to present the commendation certificate and personally thank the blood donor.
* Special privileges were offered to donors at the blood bank. The emphasis was on speed, courtesy, and professional touch combined with personal care.

(G) Politics: Sanjeevani's management appreciated that 'politics' in its positive sense is a 'game of power'. It meant using different sources of power to achieve its stated objectives. It involved:

★ Using the 'knowledge and power' of doctors and other 'experts' to create awareness, persuade potential donors and volunteers and clear misconceptions.
★ Using the 'power position' of heads of institutions, community leaders, Rotary presidents and local officials in motivating potential donors, volunteers and facilitators.
★ Using the power of 'incentives/rewards'—both monetary and non-monetary—namely, commendation certificates and gifts sponsored by facilitating organisations.
★ Using 'charisma power' of local social leaders.
★ Using 'relationship power' with frequent donors, volunteers and facilitators to get things done.

(H) Pace (speed, responsiveness): Over the years, Sanjeevani had realised that most of its clients were short of time. They expected quick and effective response. By simplifying procedures, using computers and retrievable data bases and continuous training of its personnel, Sanjeevani improved its pace of dealing with clients and this was continuously being monitored and upgraded.

2.4 LESSONS TO BE LEARNT

What can be learnt from the Sanjeevani example is summarised here:

■ CASM can succeed only if it is based on relevant and reliable culturally-adapted social market research (CASOMAR).
■ Situation analyses (SWOT)
  • CASM planners need to know their associates and competitors, their clients and the environment in which they are operating.
  • Strengths and weaknesses are internal to the organisation and opportunities and threats come from clients, competitors, associates and the environment.
  • The end product of this exercise would be quantification of opportunities and delineation of major concerns/issues for tapping these opportunities. This exercise has to be done keeping in mind the broad activities and purpose of the organisation.
■ Situation analyses should lead to a statement of short-term and long-term objectives, both quantitative and qualitative.
■ Keeping in mind its objectives, resources and characteristics and the needs of the client group, the organisation has to focus CASM on specific groups to avoid wastage of resources. They should focus on the target clients within geographical proximity whose characteristics are fairly homogeneous. This is a must to ensure that efforts are not dissipated. Target clients include both internal (its own personnel) and external clients (such as end-users, influencers and facilitators).
■ Having identified the target clients, the organisation has to decide what kind of image and relationship/interaction it would like to have vis-à-vis these client groups. This is a crucial decision. It guides the development of the CASM-mix.
■ All the activities that organisations undertake to achieve their objectives, desired image and relationships with different client groups can be broadly classified under the following 8Ps: i) Product ii) Place iii) Price iv) Promotion v) People vi) Process vii) Politics and viii) Pace.

These various considerations have to be blended properly, keeping the cultural context in mind, to achieve CASM objectives.

2.5 WHAT GOOD DOES IT DO DEVELOPERS TO UNDERSTAND CASM?

Understanding CASM helps in the diagnosis of problems that occur in the conduct of development projects. CASM helps in planning in a systematic manner. It also helps in implementing projects effectively and efficiently. However, it does not guarantee success. The major advantage of doing things systematically is that the factors responsible for success/failure can be readily identified. Cultural adaptation also helps in relating to the client groups better and more meaningfully.

2.6 WHO SHOULD CONDUCT CASM?

The options available in this regard are:

- An 'in-house CASM cluster' (mainly useful for large government departments, major donor agencies and large NGOs).
- Contract with appropriate expert agencies (attractive for medium-sized organisations with frequent CASM needs).
- Contract with specific individual professionals (similar as above). If the professional is selected with proper scrutiny, this option works out to be cheaper and more effective. But, as these professionals lack infrastructural support, the organisations availing of this option have to provide field personnel and other support to them.
- Own Staff: this applies mainly to small NGOs, where the chief executive or senior partner can undergo CASM training and act as an internal resource person. For many small NGOs, this may be the only viable option.

However, for both donor agencies and NGOs, capability building for CASM and supplementing these capabilities should be a priority.

2.7 WHAT SHOULD BE THE CASM BUDGET?

There are a number of options to consider:

- Some fixed percentage of the total budget.
- A fixed percentage higher or lower than the previous year's budget.
- By 'objective and task'. Though it is difficult to operationalise, it makes a lot of managerial sense. It simply means deciding on the objectives, then deciding on the tasks involved and finally working out the budget for the performance of those tasks. If the costs appear not to be affordable then objectives need to be modified and tasks reworked.

When preparing a CASM budget social marketers should always consider the following:

- Sensitivity of financial donors to the CASM budget.
- Basic appreciation of the importance of CASM.
- Appreciation of the fact that every CASM budget has a lower and upper threshold limit. Expenditure below the threshold limit goes waste because it may not have any impact and expenditure above the threshold level doesn't contribute incrementally.

2.8 HOW CAN CASM BE REVIEWED?

There are different procedures that can be followed. The one chosen by Sanjeevani's trustees is described here:

- A simple **one-page questionnaire** was to be administered to blood donors at the site, after their donation, to find out about their experience and elicit their suggestions on specific subjects.
- **Number of donors and volume of blood** collected at the camp sites and on the premises were to be monitored on a monthly basis to analyse trends.
- Weekly **meetings** with the regular personnel, fortnightly meetings and quarterly meetings with client institutions were planned to seek their suggestions to improve the service and seek their further commitment.

2.9 RECOMMENDED READING

Kotler, P. and **E.L. Roberto** (1989). *Social Marketing: Strategies for Changing Public Behaviour*, The Free Press, New York.

Parasuraman, A. et al. (1985). 'A Conceptual Model of Service Quality and its Implication for Future Research', *Journal of Marketing*, 49, pp. 41–50.

Peter T.J. and **J.H. Waterman Jr.** (1982). *In Search of Excellence*, Harper and Row, New York.

Wiebe, G.D. (1951–52). 'Merchandising Commodities and Citizenship on Television', *Public Opinion Quarterly*, 15, Winter pp. 679–91.

Chapter 3

Culturally-adapted Social Market Research (CASOMAR): An Essential Part of CASM

T. Scarlett Epstein

3.1   WHAT IS CASOMAR?

CASOMAR is an integral part of every CASM. It constitutes a project-specific, action-driven and action-oriented, audience-focused research. The emphasis on cultural-adaptation distinguishes it from commercial market research and its cost- and time-effectiveness as well as its interdisciplinarity distinguishes it from most social science research—in particular those conducted by most university staff and students.

CASOMAR necessitates that at least one or two of those who organise it are members of the project directorate rather than outside evaluators. This facilitates the raising and answering of questions that are specific to the project undertaken and will effectively improve its efficiency.

CASOMAR should ideally be conducted at each of the three major project phases:

3.1.1   Formative CASOMAR

This is the most important CASOMAR. It takes place at the **design phase** to establish:

- Who should the project target?
- What needs to be done?
- What indicators will be used to evaluate results?
- What are the benefits to be derived by the targeted population and do they perceive them as such?
- What image should the communication convey?

Answers to these questions must be sought not only in qualitative but also in quantitative terms. It is not enough to know **what** misconceptions people hold but also **how many** people are involved.

3.1.2   Process CASOMAR

This takes place during the **implementation phase** to monitor the ongoing project performance; it asks the following questions:

- Is the project proceeding according to plan?
- What messages have been conveyed, to whom, through what venues and by what means?
- What is the optimal mix of advertising, media promotion, public relations, and inter-personal contact?

3.1.3   Accountability CASOMAR

This takes place during the **final project phase** and evaluates the outcome and impact; it seeks answers to:

- What was the project expected to achieve?
- What were the measures used?
- Did it achieve its objectives?
- If it did not do so, why did it fail? and most important of all:
- **What, if anything could be done better?**

It is important always to remember that unlike academic studies, CASOMAR is project-focused and action-oriented; its objective is to yield information that will help ensure the success of a project, rather than to provide general knowledge.

3.2   HOW IS A CASOMAR CONDUCTED?[1]

A CASOMAR is usually divided into three stages:

3.2.1   Stage 1: Secondary Data Collection

This involves:

- Defining the problem addressed and the project objectives to provide the basis for meaningful monitoring and evaluation.
- Exploring relevant preconceptions among all those participating in the project.
- Compiling an effective data bank of all available relevant data to avoid unnecessary duplication of information.
- Preparing a CASOMAR plan by prioritising required data into those that are essential, desirable, useful, interesting but not necessary.

[1]For more detailed guidelines on how to conduct a CASOMAR see T. Scarlett Epstein et al. (1991). The earlier name used for CASOMAR was Development Market Research (DMR).

3.2.2 Stage 2: Primary Data Collection

This involves:

a) **Qualitative field research** which is primarily **exploratory and interpretative** rather than descriptive and involves relatively small numbers of people. It is an effective means to understand people's motivations and attitudes and to gain insight into people's subjective perceptions, their deep-rooted beliefs and feelings. The first task of qualitative research is to compile a cultural profile (see Chapter 4) of the selected target group. It is essential to use only **indigenous researchers for the collection of qualitative materials**; to collect such data researchers have to be tuned into the local cultural wave-length. Major methods used in qualitative research are:

- **The individual-depth-interview (IDI),** which is most effective if the enquiry deals with sensitive issues or when it is subject to peer pressure. It may also be used as a preliminary to focus group discussions (FGDs) to test the appropriateness of a discussion guide.
- **Focus group discussions** (FGDs) are held by a skilled moderator according to a tested discussion guide with selected participants, who number between four to ten depending on the topic discussed. The composition of a FGD should be as homogenous as possible in terms of age, gender, socio-economic rank.

Besides **observation,** qualitative research also uses a number of projective enquiry techniques, of which the major ones are listed here:

- **Role play** which usually entails respondents acting out their perceptions of an idea or service; this is particularly effective if among the FGD members there can be found a few extrovert individuals with acting abilities. For example, role play was successfully used in a CASOMAR that examined the effectiveness of a community health service. When two FGD participants were asked to act out how the community health worker related to individuals in the community, it quickly emerged that the group perceived it as a top-down authoritarian relationship. The man playing the part of the health worker sat himself down on a bench and a woman with her head bent in an obedient fashion approached him. She requested his help and advice for her complaint in response to which the official shouted his orders in an authoritarian fashion. The rest of the group watched the performance with great interest; they all nodded in agreement and enthusiastically applauded at the end of it. This clearly indicated that the community felt that the health worker behaved in a dictatorial rather than in a helpful manner. Whether or not the health worker really behaved in this manner was not really important—what mattered was how his behaviour was perceived.
- **Association,** which includes word association and spontaneous association, often clearly indicates people's true feelings and perceptions. This technique can be used as part of IDIs and/or FGDs. For example, when an interviewer aimed to discover what a female informant thought about joining a proposed income-generating project and asked her what immediately came to her mind, she spontaneously uttered 'violence'. When this was further explored with her, it emerged that her husband threatened to beat the life out of her if she earned money without handing it over to him. She would never have been prepared to reveal this in the course of an ordinary interview.

- **Sentence completion** involves the moderator asking respondents to complete sentences. If the object of the CASOMAR is to find out prevailing attitudes regarding family planning, it is unlikely that a straight-forward question such as 'What do you think about family planning' would produce reliable and truthful answers. Everyone these days knows that they are expected to have no more than two children and people are always inclined to give the answer they think is expected of them. By using the technique of sentence completion, however, the moderator may find out about actual attitudes to family planning. The respondents are asked to complete the sentence 'A woman who has 10 children is...'. If they add 'a good wife' it clearly indicates that they approve of a woman having many children; if on the other hand they complete the sentence with the word 'crazy', it shows their interest in the use of contraceptives.
- **A person from outer space** is another technique used. Respondents are asked to imagine that a person from outer space, completely ignorant of the subject under discussion, is present and are then asked to describe it to the aliens. This technique is particularly useful if in the course of the FGD the moderator notices that group members are reluctant to speak out freely because they assume that the moderator already knows all the answers. A person from outer space obviously cannot be expected to know anything of what has been going on and this often helps to remove people's barriers to articulate their thoughts.
- **Obituaries** entails respondents describing a product or service as if it had died. What were its advantages and its weaknesses; how could it have made its life better? This is a useful device to find out what respondents really think about the matter under discussion and, what is even more important, to discover how they perceive it may be improved.
- **Photo sorting** entails respondents selecting from a large number of photographs those which they consider best reflect their perception of the subject under discussion; this too can be very revealing of respondents' real thoughts on the subject matter.

The analysis of the collected qualitative data helps to form the basis for a succinct questionnaire survey to provide quantitative materials. However, it must be mentioned here that many social science professionals have become disenchanted with questionnaire surveys simply because these enquiries are conducted in a highly artificial situation. The critics complain that in a questionnaire survey 'you have an interviewer asking very specific questions of a stranger who has given almost no previous thought to what he is being questioned about. The subject winds up giving the answers he thinks he is supposed to give. The results can be expressed in neat percentages, but as a practical matter they are mostly useless'. Yet quantified data are still crucial for policy-makers who have to decide between alternative policy choices. To counterbalance the disadvantages of both qualitative and quantitative research, an effective CASOMAR has to pursue both in a complementary fashion.

b) **Quantitative Research** by contrast with its qualitative counterpart is characterised by the following criteria:

- **It focuses on large numbers of people**, considered as the 'universe'.
- **It selects a sample** (a smaller portion of the universe) usually by means of one of the many random sampling procedures.
- **It uses a structured questionnaire with pre-coded answers**, which is pilot tested.
- **It analyses the results statistically often with the help of computers**, and presents them in the form of tables.

- **It facilitates the generalisation of results over the total universe**. Before general-ising, however, it is advisable to validate and verify the results of the sample survey.

The role of the interviewer is crucial in CASOMAR. Therefore, interviewers must be carefully trained, briefed on each specific project in which they are engaged and put through field tests. Strict supervision must be exercised over their work. It is advantageous to process completed questionnaires while the survey is still going on to spot shortcomings before it is too late to change the survey procedures.

3.2.3   Stage 3: Processing of Qualitative Data and Preparation of a CASOMAR Report

The processing of qualitative data involves:

- **Transcription/translation** of tapes and/or notes that have been recorded in the course of FGDs and IDIs. Transcription should be verbatim and translation as accurate as possible.
- **Coding and analysis:** Coding usually involves a preliminary analysis. The full-blown analysis focuses on interpreting the collected information and to explain its meaning.
- **The report** combines the findings of the secondary data investigation and the qualitative and quantitative research. The qualitative section usually contains relevant verbatim quotations of respondents to illustrate the language actually used. The report is usually structured into five sections:

  - ★ **Executive summary** which presents conclusions and recommendations in bullet format.
  - ★ **Background and introduction** which spells out the research brief and gives details of the research methodology and techniques used.
  - ★ **Findings and recommendations** which present the major findings and provide action-oriented recommendations. It constitutes the most important part of the report.
  - ★ **Content analysis** which contains an analytical presentation and discussion of research findings.
  - ★ **Appendices** that include tables, copies of the discussion guide, questionnaires and stim-ulus materials used.

- **Presentation of report** is the occasion when the researchers discuss with the project directorate their prepared report. The object of this exercise is to provide sufficient information at this stage, to facilitate immediate action to be taken based on the recommendations.

3.3   WHO CAN ORGANISE CASOMAR?

CASOMAR can be organised by:

- ■ **In-house arrangements** as part of existing organisational structures. For instance, a number of ministries—e.g., the Ministries of Health, Social Welfare and Rural Development—may jointly set up a CASOMAR section that uses their existing appropriate office and field staff to collect, process and analyse CASOMAR data. Their research can be conducted in an **omnibus** fashion, which yields the advantages of economies of scale.

■ **Specialised agencies** can be contracted to conduct specific CASOMAR, by NGOs, most of whom are too small to have their in-house arrangements. Such agencies provide efficient service, but may be too costly for small NGOs.

■ **Experts in market research**, many of whom are often pleased to help a laudable cause in a voluntary capacity, can train and work together with existing NGO staff.

3.4   HOW LONG DOES A CASOMAR TAKE?

The time a CASOMAR takes will obviously vary with different projects; it may take as little as one month or as much as five months, depending on the type of problem tackled and the information sought. In any case it is important that time and expenditure is budgeted at the outset of each CASOMAR.

3.5   CAN THE COST OF CASOMAR BE JUSTIFIED?

CASOMAR is a worthwhile and highly cost-effective investment. Though it increases project expenditure, it considerably reduces wastage of resources in the long-term by improving project efficiency and increasing the chances of sustainability.

3.6   RECOMMENDED READING

Balch, G.I. and **M.S. Sutton** (1997). 'Keep Me Posted: A Plea for Practical Evaluation' in M.E. Goldberg et al. (eds), *Social Marketing—Theoretical and Practical Perspectives*, Lawrence Erlbaum Associates, London.

Cronbach, I.J. (1982). *Designing Evaluations and Social Programs*, Jossey-Bass, San Francisco.

Epstein, T. Scarlett et al. (1991). *A Training Manual for Development Market Research Investigators*, BBC World Service, London.

Epstein, T. Scarlett (1995). *Improving NGO Development Programs—Proceedings of the Training Workshop on Culturally-Adapted Development Market Research (CADMR)*, CARD Foundation, Manila.

Mytton, Graham (forthcoming). Handbook on Media and Audience Research, UNICEF and BBC, New York and London.

Patton, M.Q. (1986). *Utilization-focused Evaluation* (2nd. edn.), DDB Needham Worldwide, Chicago.

———— (1990). *Qualitative Evaluation and Research Methods* (2nd. edn.), Sage, Newbury Park, CA.

Chapter 4

The Cultural-adaptation of Social Market Research and Social Marketing[1]

T. Scarlett Epstein

Market research and marketing originated in the industrialised societies of Western Europe and North America. These commercial practices therefore have a specific *a priori* cultural bias. This is, for instance, symbolised in the emphasis placed on the views of individual respondents, which is in tune with the value these industrial cultures attach to individual decision-making. By contrast, many other cultures practise group rather than individual decision-making. Therefore, market enquiries have to be adapted accordingly to ensure meaningful results. Such cultural adaptation is of even greater importance in the context of social market research and social marketing. This is so because the success of many development projects depends on changes in social behaviour that are often deeply rooted in traditional cultural norms—without an understanding of which it is unlikely that the necessary and socially desirable behavioural changes can ever be expected to take place.

4.1   THE IMPORTANT ROLE OF CULTURE

Each society has its own traditional culture which includes behavioural norms and an inventory of solutions. In order to survive, collectivities have over the generations had to develop a system of solutions to deal with the problems arising out of their natural and social environment. For instance, since high infant mortality threatened group survival most 'cultural inventories of solutions' include magical measures to ensure the continuity of the collectivity such as guidelines to what a barren woman should do so that she may bear children, or how to protect the health of a new-born child. Most societies, previously, never faced any threat to their survival from having too many children. Therefore the traditional 'cultural inventories of solutions' do not include guidelines of how to deal with this problem. This can account for the fact that it takes many years for fertility changes to occur.

[1] For a detailed discussion of why and how social market research and social marketing need to be culturally-adapted refer to Recommended reading, Epstein, T. Scarlett (1988), (1993), (1997).

Many developers fail to understand local cultures. They expect Third World societies to adopt new behavioural patterns as if there existed no traditional norms. A common fallacy, particularly among 'scientific' health professionals, may be described by altering the biblical parable of the old wine and the new. The vessels in this instance are the clients of health action, and one cannot exchange them for new ones. Medical workers, who wish to pour the new wine of scientific ideas into these vessels, often forget that they are not empty. Popular health culture is the wine that fills them, and ignoring this often results in spilling the new wine on the ground. Thus one may refer to the *fallacy of the empty vessels.* interesting.

4.1.1   How are Individual Cultures Perpetuated?

Each individual is **socialised** into the norms of its society even before reaching the age of five i.e., before formal schooling starts!. Children are taught the Do's and Don'ts of their culture: they learn how to speak, how to eat, are toilet trained etc. In other words, the cultural inventory of solutions is passed on to succeeding generations at a very early stage in their lives, to prepare them to face the problems that they are likely to encounter. To ensure lasting behavioural changes in tune with changing environmental conditions, it is normally necessary to change the messages that are passed on to succeeding generations in the course of their socialisation. This helps to explain why it usually takes more than one generation before new problems are tackled.

4.1.2   Who does the Socialising?

To introduce a change in the content of socialisation it is essential to discover **WHO** socialises infants in the target society. In Western industrialised societies where the nuclear family has become the norm, infants are taken care of by their own mother, father, and/or a childminder. Among many Third World societies there still exist three generation families—i.e., grandparents live with one or more of their married children and their unmarried grandchildren. It is usually the grandmother who socialises her grandchildren while the mother is away at work. A lack of appreciation of the importance of grandmothers in ensuring behavioural changes has lead to the failure of numerous public health projects. For instance, the world-wide child immunisation campaign in many places failed to identify grandmothers as the chief childminders and *a priori* took young mothers as their exclusive target. However, the immunisation publicity did not reach the young women who were often busy working away from home all day while their children were being cared for by their grandmothers. No attempt was made to alert grandmothers about the desirability of protecting infants against infectious diseases. As a result many children failed to be immunised.

4.1.3   Why Many Developers Still Ignore the Impact of Culture

Most agencies concerned with the different aspects of development concentrate on hiring technical expertise related to the field of their intervention. For instance, a nutritional project will hire nutritionists and food engineers. A social scientist, who would ensure that due emphasis is given to the cultural background into which the project has to fit, is seldom hired. Yet before a technical expert can be expected to effect changes in behavioural patterns and therefore, cultural norms, it is essential that s/he understands the relevant aspects of the existing cultural norms and their rationale.

4.1.4   How Culture can be Identified

The lack of cost- and time-effective methods to investigate the impact of cultural factors appears to have been the major reason why developers of all kinds and even market researchers have tended to overlook the strategic role of culture.

Until not so long ago, the compilation of cultural profiles had been the prerogative of social anthropologists, whose in-depth micro-society studies usually take a number of years and are therefore costly and not of much practical use to developers and planners. However, social market researchers and social marketers in particular have, in the course of their activities, come to appreciate the need for reliable cost- and time-effective information on the different cultures of their various target societies. For social marketing to be effective its target has to be culturally homogenous; careful target segmentation is essential. This has resulted in the emergence of some cost- and time-effective methods to discover why targeted groups behave the way they do; a few of the most important of these methods are outlined below:

4.1.4.1   *Lifestyle Studies*

These are based on relatively rudimentary demographic data extracted from census data and other secondary source material readily available in Western industrialised countries and are used widely in the context of target segmentation. The difficulty with using lifestyle studies in Third World countries is that first, there is often a lack of relevant official up-to-date statistics and those that are available may not be accurate. Second, official statistics provide only superficial information about the selected target audience. For example, the data tell us only that the target audience are women 18 to 45 years old living in major metropolises with their husbands and having at least one child under age five. This secondary data gives no insight into the behavioural patterns of target societies, what their needs, wants, aspirations and perceptions really are.

4.1.4.2   *Activities, Interest, and Opinion (AIO) Studies*

These try to remedy the deficiencies of lifestyle studies by collecting detailed qualitative motivation information from probability sampled households and then clusters target audiences into groups similar in AIO profiles. Such lifestyle profiles yield rich insights into the target audience's particular interests, media habits, leisure patterns and so on. These insights are very valuable in formulating messages that effectively address specific target audiences. This type of research, however, seems to work well only with upper strata Western audiences. It is far more difficult to use AIO methods in studying the social behaviour of the poorest people who are the target of many Third World development projects.

4.1.4.3   *Project-specific Key Cultural Variables (KCVs)*

These constitute a means to compile cost- and time-effective cultural profiles of Third World target societies. The KCV concept represents a compromise between reliance on what are frequently unsatisfactory official statistics and alien and/or quick questionnaire surveys on the one hand and the lengthy and costly anthropological studies on the other. KCVs use anthropological insight in a developmental context to ensure that projects are culture-sensitive: They are thus action-oriented. The well-tried and efficient qualitative methods and techniques which have been developed in the context of commercial market research are used in exploring how the project-specific KCVs operate among the selected target societies. The use of project-specific KCVs facilitates the compilation of a target group's cultural profile within a few days! It should be stressed here though that such cultural profiles will be more superficial and not as reliable as the lengthy micro-studies conducted by professional anthropologists.

However, for practical purposes, the KCV-based cultural profiles suffice for at least ensuring cultural sensitivity relating to projects in general and social marketing in particular. As project-specific KCVs seem to constitute the most appropriate method available to date, that ensures that social marketing is culturally-adapted, I give a summary of how KCVs can be used in the context of different projects here.

4.2 HOW CAN PROJECT-SPECIFIC KCV DATA BE COLLECTED?

Project-specificity means that the KCVs investigated will be different for different projects. The first task is to compile a list of project-specific KCVs.

4.2.1 Project-specific Lists of KCVs

The compilation of project-specific lists of KCVs does not necessarily have to be done by qualified social scientists—though it is an advantage if it can be done by one. But, a staff member, with field experience and some social science training, is usually able to prepare a list of KCVs that effectively helps to provide a cultural profile of the target society. To illustrate the different types of KCVs that are appropriate for different projects, two examples of KCV lists that have been used in specific projects are given here:

4.2.1.1   *A Nutrition Project*

A Project to improve the Nutrition of Pregnant and Lactating Women:

Unit of decision-making	Role models
Income-generating resources	Prestige criteria
Socialisers and content of socialisation	Religious beliefs
Food taboos	Nutrition folklore

In this nutrition project a familiarity with existing food taboos and relevant folklore besides the more general cultural variables was essential to introduce nutritional improvements. The data for the cultural profile was collected in the course of three IDIs of one grandmother and one each of a young mother and her husband, as well as an FGD composed of grandmothers and another of young married women. The resulting information indicated that: The three generation joint family acts as one decision-making unit; young couples settle with the husband's parents where his mother passes onto her grandchildren the traditional cultural norms, which include food taboos including what are defined as 'hot food' items such as e.g., bananas; abstinence is considered as a main prestige criteria and religious beliefs are rather fundamentalist with religious functionaries being regarded as role models; rice cultivation is the main source of subsistence and income. On the basis of this cultural profile the social marketing segmented the target into: a) religious functionaries, b) grandmothers, c) young married women and d) their husbands. For each of these targets, different communication strategies were used to convince them of the advantages of the nutritional changes proposed for pregnant and lactating women.

Role Model

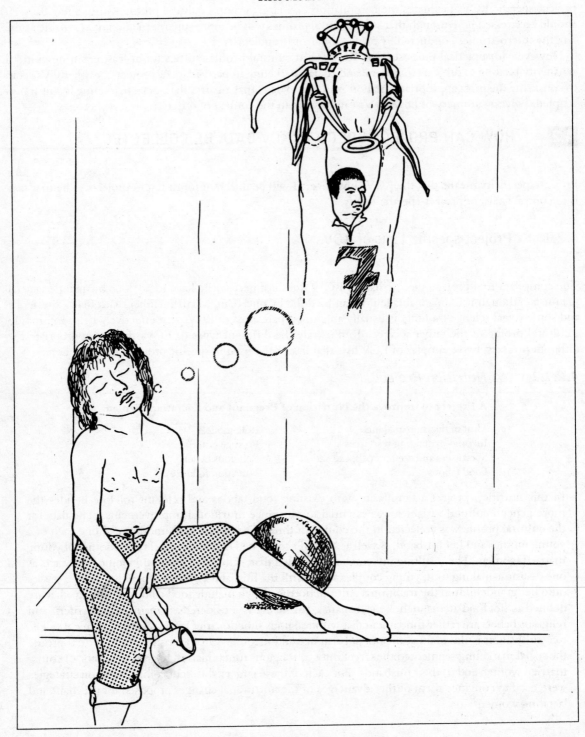

Gender Relations

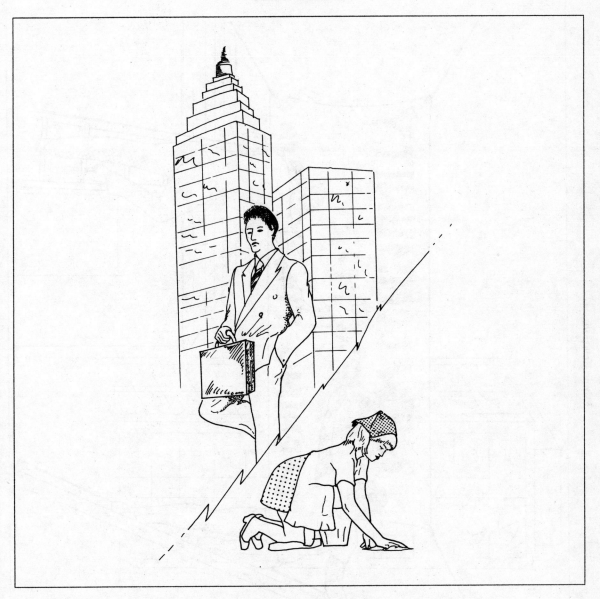

A Reproductive Health Project

Unit of decision-making
Socialisers and content of socialisation
Gender relations
Son preference
Privacy

Sexual mores
Religious beliefs
Prestige criteria
Ethnic relations
Economic activities

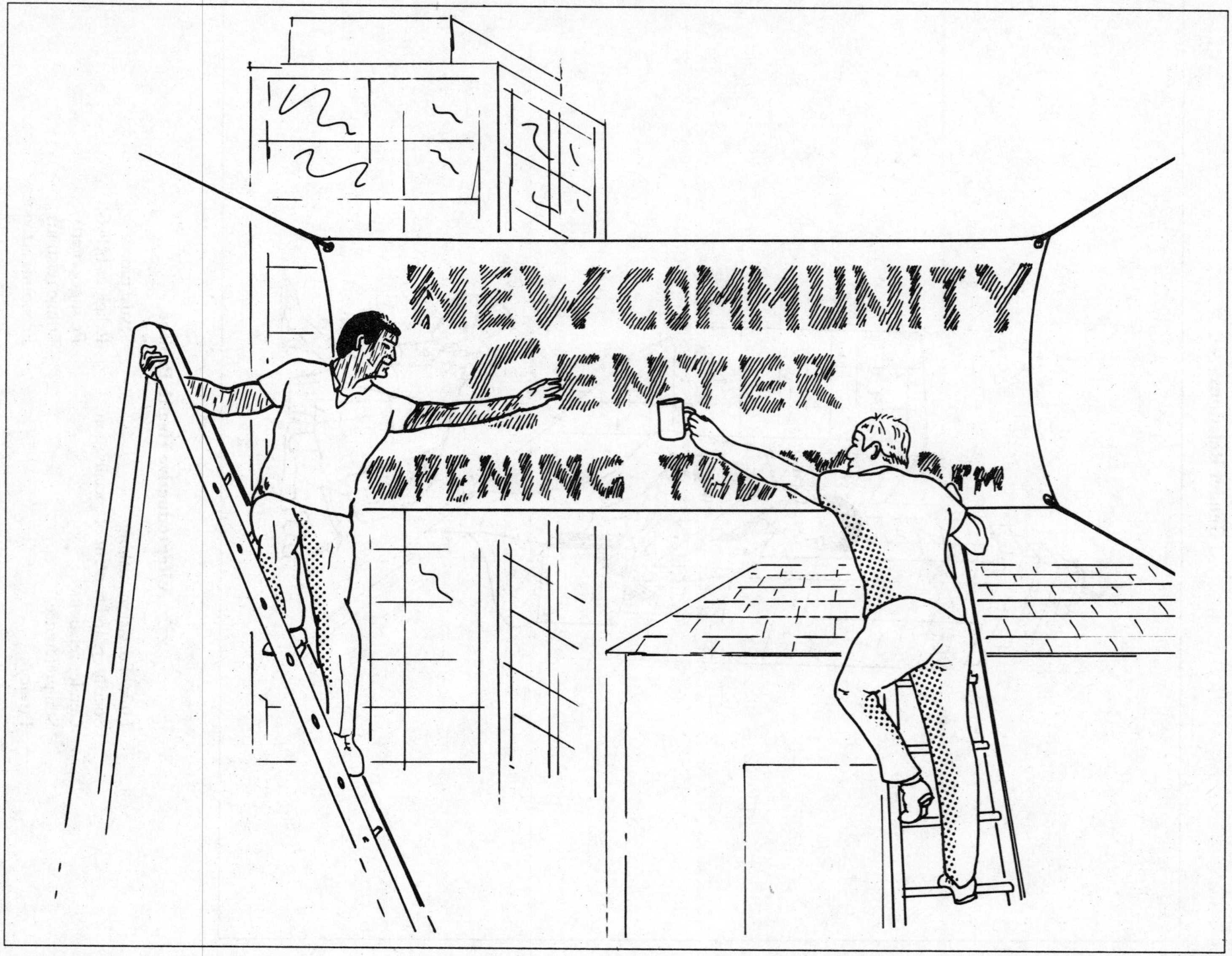
NEW COMMUNITY
CENTER
OPENING TO

It was decided that for the reproductive health project to succeed it needed to be based on a sound understanding of the influence on reproductive behaviour exerted by the existing sexual mores, son preference, religious beliefs, how and by whom these cultural norms were being perpetuated and the overall economic setting. Two IDIs (one with a grandmother and another with a young married woman) as well as four FGDs (one composed of grandmothers, another of women in their reproductive age, a third of married men and a fourth of male high school students) were organised to elicit the required information. The research indicated that it was taboo for a mother to talk about sex with her daughter; it was the responsibility of the grandmother to initiate her grand-daughters into the traditional sexual mores which stressed son preference and the need to have many children to ensure prestige and counterbalance high infant mortality; the majority of the population were Catholics and local priests threatened to excommunicate all those who ventured to use contraceptives; couples had little privacy and young wives were afraid to discuss reproductive health with anyone except their group of female peers—they would not talk about sexual matters even with their own husbands; economic activities were all strictly gender-specific and men were considered the main providers who had a right to expect their wives to bear as many children as possible. On the basis of this information the target society was, for purposes of social marketing, divided into six homogenous segmentss: a) grandmothers, b) women in their reproductive age, c) married men, d) male adolescents, e) female adolescents, f) Roman Catholic priests. For each of these segments different communication strategies were used.

4.2.2 Methods used to Establish how the Selected KCVs Operate in the Target Society

In addition to the methods already discussed (see 3.2.2), local school teachers may be encouraged to get their pupils to write essays on project-relevant cultural topics. These essays can help to throw a lot of light on the local cultural norms and practices.

I hope that the preceding presentation will convince readers that:

The effectiveness of social market researchers and social marketers will be greatly enhanced if they are tuned into the cultures of their different target societies and that this in turn will be reflected in an increased success rate of development projects.

4.3 RECOMMENDED READING

Balch, G.I. and **S.M. Sutton** (1997). 'Keep Me Posted—A Plea for Practical Evaluation' in M.E. Goldberg et al. (eds), *Social Marketing—Theoretical and Practical Perspectives*, Lawrence Erlbaum Associates, London.

Epstein, T. Scarlett (1988). *A Manual for Culturally-Adapted Market Research in the Development Process*, RWAL Publications, Sussex.

———— (1993). 'Development Market Research: Client-led versus Top-down Development', *Project Appraisal*, March.

———— (1997). 'Safe Motherhood—Appropriate Communication Methods and Techniques', *Action for Safe Motherhood (UK), Newsletter No. 8*.

Green, L.W. and **M.W. Kreuter** (1991). *Health Promotion Planning: An Educational and Environmental Approach*, Mayfield, Mountain View, CA.

Sutton, S.M. (1992). 'Evaluation Research: Opportunity or Obstacle to Good Communications' in *Proceedings: Evaluation Research*, Office of Disease Prevention and Health Promotion, U.S. Dept. of Health and Human Services, Washington, DC.

Chapter 5

How does CASM Communicate and Publicise its Messages?

Mithileshwar Jha

A seasoned bureaucrat was sitting through a public meeting in a remote tribal area in India. Several extension experts, environmental experts and forest officials gave very stimulating lectures to the tribal audience on the importance of conservation of forests in a language that they could understand, but with little observable impact. When his turn came, he simply lifted the glass of water standing in front of him. Then, he called a young tribal boy with thick curly hair, from the audience.

The audience looked on with excitement. He first dropped some water on his own bald head. Every drop fell down, to the delight of the audience. Then he poured some water on the thick curly hair of the tribal boy. Some of the water fell down, but some of it remained even when the boy shook his head. He then drew an analogy of barren hills with his bald head, and that of land covered with thick forests with the thick curly hair of the boy. The audience gave an appreciating nod. He didn't have to preach to the tribals about the value of water and conservation.

A professional advertising agency tried to develop a campaign to remind mothers with new born babies about the booster dosage of polio drops and the triple antigen vaccine to protect the child against polio, and diphtheria pertusis and tetanus. In a rural setting, with a very low level of female literacy rate, the task was difficult. However, while visiting rural homes, a researcher from the agency came across 'almanacs' (calendars which mention auspicious days and timings based on certain astrological calculations). The researcher also discovered that these almanacs were preserved and consulted periodically during the year. Based on this, the agency prepared its own almanac with a focus on vaccine booster dosage and messages regarding child and mother health care (the almanac also contained the regular information).

These are a few of the several imaginative, culturally-adapted social communications which are simple and effective. However, there is no dearth of counter examples also. One often hears dedicated personnel of social service organisations making statements like:

'People are their own enemies. We tried our best, but they never listen'.

'So much of our resources and efforts are wasted on educating and convincing people, that there is little left for the actual task'.

'We have tried to educate the people; it depends on them how they use it'.

These examples highlight the complexity of CASM communication. The major steps involved and the critical issues for each step are outlined in Table 5.1.

Table 5.1
Steps and Issues Involved in the CASM Communication/Promotion Process

Serial Number	Steps	Issues	Reference* Paragraph
1.	Deciding the **target audience**	1.1 Who should be the target audience? 1.2 What should we know about the target audience? 1.3 How do we develop an understanding of the target audience?	5.1
2.	Defining the **communication/ promotion objectives**	2.1 Why should we be clear about the objectives? 2.2 How do we define objectives?	5.2
3.	Deciding the **communication-mix**	3.1 What are the elements of a communication-mix? 3.2 When do we use one element and when the other? 3.3 How do we combine these for greater effectiveness?	5.3
4.	Deciding on the **message**	4.1 What should we say, to whom? 4.2 How should we say it?	5.4
5.	Deciding the **media and its schedule**	5.1 What are the media options available for CASM? 5.2 How do we select an option or a combination of options? 5.3 How frequently do we use different media?	5.5
6.	Deciding the **media budget**	6.1 How do we decide how much is adequate?	5.6
7.	**Reviewing CASM communication/promotion** decisions	7.1 What and how do we review? 7.2 How do we keep communicating more effectively and efficiently?	5.7

*Refers to paragraphs where the issues are discussed

The issues raised in relation to each step are briefly discussed here:

5.1   DECIDING ON THE TARGET AUDIENCE

This is a key decision in the CASM communication/promotion-mix. The purpose of communication is to get a response. For this we need to know what response we want, from whom, what is the current predisposition of our target audience; why, and so on.

5.1.1   Who should be the Target Audience?

Development professionals deal with multiple audiences. For example, in Case Study D (CASM for HIV/AIDS/STDs—A Community Self-Help Programme in Kenya) 'out-of-school and socially apart youth' are identified as the target audience for messages and help. The youth themselves are a heterogenous group consisting of street vendors, dormitory supervisors, night porters at clinics, clergy members and sex workers.

It helps to identify the major client groups, their specific role in a situation, main actors within these groups and their relevant motivations. For example, we need to understand what type of street vendors would be interested in participating in a programme for AIDS prevention? How can they be involved? What could be their role? What would be the best way to enroll them and to ensure their continuing involvement with the programme?

We need to identify opinion leaders and other influential persons or facilitators (see Chapter 2 for examples from the blood donor project). It is crucial for the success of the programmes, to reduce the public into as many target clients as possible. Target clients cannot easily be identified through normal observations. For example, only through an insightful CASOMAR could the role played by grandmothers and elder siblings in the day-to-day care of infants and children in developing countries be highlighted. However, one should not try to diffuse one's attention over too many target audiences. Development organisations, with limited resources and complex issues, need to **focus** their attention on **key** target audiences.

5.1.2   What do We Need to Know about our Target Audiences?

We need to know as much about our target audience as possible. The examples at the beginning of this chapter and the various case studies included in this manual emphasise this. Specifically we need to know the following:

- Their current predispositions and motivations, their geographic (area and locality of stay), demographic (age, sex, income, profession, education and literacy), psychographic (attitudes, interests, opinions on relevant issues and lifestyle), behaviouristic (what kinds of relevant activities do they currently indulge in; do they demonstrate loyalty to certain charities and so on) background and media habits (like, newspapers, magazines read regularly, television and radio programmes viewed/listened to and films seen).
- Their roles and status in society, as seen by the audience groups and as perceived by others. For example, many professional physicians working in rural India initially showed disdain for local *dais* (traditional midwives) but after understanding their status among women, they began to see them as important individuals and used them as essential links in mother and child welfare programmes.
- The norms, symbols, key words and gestures used, and their prior experience.
- How are the developers themselves perceived by the target audience. For example, the response of HIV patients to the publicity which they perceive originates from do-gooders may be completely different compared to publicity channeled to them through their own friends.

5.1.3   How do We Gain an Understanding of our Target Audience?

This requires frequent interaction, staying together for long periods, participation in their daily lives and rituals, and building trust-based relationships. It also requires listening skills, social skills and empathy.

Initial understanding could be developed through various CASOMAR methods using psychological research techniques like role play, sentence completion and story writing. It should then be developed and nurtured as mentioned earlier.

5.2 DECIDING ON THE COMMUNICATION/PROMOTION OBJECTIVES

5.2.1 Why should We be Clear about Objectives?

Many development professionals think and feel that in any development situation there are multiple objectives. Hence, it's neither prudent nor possible to develop clarity on objectives. The focus is on action—to get going, with the view that something will be achieved. However, this is a faulty strategy and the following need to be appreciated:

- Development communication objectives can vary from **just creating awareness to behavioural changes**.
- Appropriate approaches, resources and efforts required for these two extremes vary considerably.
- It may be extremely difficult and in most cases impossible to achieve more than one objective through a single approach.
- The very process of developing clarity on objectives not only helps in focussing on important issues and in sequencing of activities, but it also helps in understanding the issues better and developing meaningful, actionable strategies. It also helps in monitoring and evaluating CASM activities.

5.2.2 How do We Define Objectives?

The purpose of communication is to seek a response from the target audience. This response could be one or more of the following:

- **Creating awareness**, e.g., making migrant labour aware of the dangers of AIDS (see Case Study D).
- **Creating knowledge**, e.g., educate the same audience about the modes of transmission of the HIV virus and possible prevention devices.
- **Developing preference/liking**, e.g., the communication may aim to develop preference/liking for use of condoms for safe sex amongst the target audience.
- **Developing conviction/behaviour-intention/behaviour** among the target audience. Mere liking/preference may not be enough where change in attitude and/or behaviour is required. For example, in the blood donation case, the liking for the cause and the organisation needs to be converted into an urge to donate and finally to the act of donating blood.

Keeping the above in mind the development professionals need to develop specific, time bound objectives (see example 2.2.2 for Sanjeevani's objectives). The communication objectives have to be derived from the overall programme objectives. One should keep in mind that good communication can help in creating awareness, knowledge and preference, but to assume that attitudes and behaviour can be changed through communication only is not being realistic.

5.3   DECISIONS ON THE COMMUNICATION-MIX

5.3.1   What are the Elements of a Communication-Mix?

The major elements of the CASM communication/promotion-mix, along with their definition and some illustrative examples, are listed in Table 5.2. A lot of myths surround social cause promotion which distracts from the reality of the beneficial impact. This is set out in Table 5.3.

5.3.2   When do We Use One Element and When the Other?

Advantages and disadvantages of different communication/promotion elements are highlighted in Table 5.4.

5.3.3   How do We Combine these for Greater Effectiveness?

The CASM communication/promotion-mix, if properly coordinated, yields superior responses compared with unsystematic and uncoordinated promotional endeavours. For example, for creating initial enthusiasm on a large scale, a combination of news releases through press interviews (publicity), advertisements in popular press, followed by some well planned events (like, children's painting competition, or sports events) may be quite effective. For converting this initial enthusiasm into specific actions, direct marketing and personal communications channels may have to be used. For small NGOs it may be desirable to approach professionals in these disciplines to provide help in planning and executing communication, either free of cost or on a token cost basis (many professionals derive immense satisfaction in working for a cause). They can also request donor agencies to separately budget for these activities, which helps in identifying and developing relationships with relevant professionals. Larger NGOs can use consultants, their own professional staff or advertising agencies for this purpose.

5.4   DECISIONS ON THE MESSAGE

5.4.1   What should We Say, to Whom?

CASM communicators face a major issue here. 'Life after cancer is worth living' attracts lots of attention. The same is true for the message 'Cancer, detected early, is curable'. But many other messages, asking people above 40 years of age to go for cancer screening, have not had much impact. Several appeals for blood donation have had no success, but the simple message 'Give blood, save life' has worked. The 'Giant Chinese Panda' as the World Wide Fund for Nature (WWF)'s symbol, makes people across the globe take positive action, some other endangered species of reptiles or crocodiles may not have that kind of impact.

Table 5.2

Elements of CASM Communication/Promotion-Mix

Serial Number	Element	Definition	Example
1.	Advertising	Any paid form of non-personal communication of products (for example, goods, services, ideas) through a commercial media by an identified sponsor.	'Life after cancer is worth living' 'Donate Blood, Save Life' Organisations like Cancer Relief Society, UNICEF, World Wide Fund for Nature (WWF) have made excellent use of advertising for creating awareness about their causes and also for generating funds. UNICEF, for example, has done this by persuading people to buy their cards. Use of the 'Panda' by WWF indicates a high degree of global cultural homogeneity of positive response for the animal. Chief Relief and You (CRY) in India has used it very effectively.
2.	Sales promotion/ incentives	These consist of various activities and incentives targeted at the end-consumers, and other customers, including the organisation's own personnel.	Activities like demonstrations, distributing samples, displaying the product or service description, participating in exhibitions and organising competitions, fall in this category. Also, providing incentives like attractive gifts for family planning adopters and persuaders, prizes, plaques for own employees, public reception of social workers, donors, facilitating bureaucrats or bankers.
3.	Cost-free publicity	Any non-paid form of media coverage.	Social cause organisations get lots of free media coverage by organising newsworthy events, inviting VIPs, writing useful topical articles and so on.
4.	Public relations	Involves managing interfaces with the relevant publics in both micro and macro environments.	Many small NGOs avail of the services of retired bureaucrats to manage positively its relationship with the donor and other relevant organisations through systematic planning of communication, personal meetings and visits.
5.	Personal selling	Involves face-to-face communication with a view to solicit a favourable response.	Selling of UNICEF cards by commission agents or volunteers. Family planning or mother and child health workers convincing women about the advantages of having a small family and to pay attention to its hygiene.
6.	Direct marketing	This is simply a marketing concept in practice. It involves developing a rich database of target respondents and approaching them directly through multiple means (for example, direct mail, telephone, personal visits) to solicit a response.	Direct mailers from various social cause organisations solicit volunteer time, donations, followed by telephone reminders or personal visits.
7.	Events marketing	This involves sponsoring and organising an event centered around a cause. Events generate a fun-filled atmosphere and excitement, which result in greater involvement and large scale responses.	Many social cause organisations arrange charity shows, walks and popular games, to create awareness and generate large amounts of donations.

Table 5.3
Myths Versus Reality about the Beneficial Impact of Social Cause Promotional Activities

Serial Number	Myths	Reality
1.	Promotion is a commercial activity to entice gullible customers.	It is a valid form of communication-persuasion process. Put to proper use, it can be very effective in getting desired responses. It can also be misused, like any other idea or item.
2.	These elements require tremendous investments.	No. Low cost alternatives are available for all the elements. For example, hand-bills or free-inserts in newspapers are low cost means of reaching sizable numbers. Newspapers and magazines do offer free or low cost space for social causes. Celebrities offer their time, if the cause is worthwhile and if they are approached in a professional manner. It also enhances their image.
3.	You need a lot of professionals and only a large organisation can do it effectively.	You need a professional approach and not numbers. Small and large professional organisations exist in almost all developed and developing countries, which provide planning and execution support.
4.	There is a sense of guilt for spending money on social market research, professional consultants, or incentives to facilitators, etc. rather than on the 'real' activity.	For achieving one's noble objectives, several tasks have to be performed. These are essential and not necessary evils. Properly done, they enhance the overall effectiveness and efficiency of the programme, resulting in more value than the costs incurred. For example, the Government of India's Family Planning Programme started in the 1950s, despite being a pioneering programme, resulted in a lot of wastage till 1970s in the absence of a well conceived CASM approach. By contrast, the child immunisation programme of GOI, conceptualised and implemented as 'Child Protection' (Shishu Suraksha) Programme used many or most of these elements, widely supported by UNICEF, and is considered a huge success.
5.	A successful thing from one situation can easily be imitated in another situation.	Innovative imitation is appreciable. However, social causes evoke deeply felt responses. They deal with attitudes, values and norms. Hence, cultural adaptation is a must. For example, economic incentives didn't help the cause of family planning in India, as was thought earlier by the planners, women's literacy helped. Open selling of contraceptives is still taboo in many countries.
6.	These are 'cosmetic' or 'peripheral' activities. Some budget may be allocated to these, if discretionary cash is available.	A minimum threshold expenditure is a must for promotion, depending on the objective and the tasks. Otherwise, the amount spent goes waste. A prime-time spot on television for *30 seconds*, if used for just one insertion per week may not even get noticed.

Table 5.4

Advantages/Disadvantages of Various CASM Communication/Promotion Elements

Serial Number	Element	Advantages	Disadvantages
1.	Advertising	* Can reach large numbers * Press advertising can put across rational messages * Television and other audiovisual media can be used for low-involvement learning and emotional appeals * Press advertisements can be preserved and re-read * Can trigger interpersonal discussion through informative and provocative messages * Effective in creating awareness and knowledge	* High initial cost * Despite databases on media habits of target audiences, lack of target segmentation often results in wastage of exposure on non-target audience * Because of proliferation of media, media planning and scheduling requires special expertise, commonly not available in social-cause organisations * Lots of messages get lost in the clutter * Not effective for inducing action
2.	Sales Promotion Incentives	* Good at inducing action * Relatively easier to measure effectiveness * Wide choice available	* Executive requires good managerial skill * Feeling of hard-sell, not conducive in many social situations * Somewhat costly
3.	Publicity	* Cheap free of cost * More easily believed as there seem to be no vested interests * Wide outreach	* Requires good networking with media and good managerial ability * Can work both ways, too much of media exposure creates suspicion and media persons also start looking for more 'news worthy' news about the organisation
4.	Public Relations	* More focused and personalised * If managed properly, it leads to active support base and participation * Enhances image at relatively lower cost among targets	* Requires good managerial input * Takes considerable time and effort * Requires lots of visits, and may at times distract from the main task * Some groups of people may have lots of nuisance value but may be difficult to exclude
5.	Personal Selling	* Personal touch * Effective in persuasive communication and in changing behaviour * Better control over outreach and variation in approach possible	* Relatively costly * It is difficult to get and retain quality sales personnel * Variations in quality of interactions is difficult to control
6.	Direct Marketing	* Very focused * Use of multiple channels can help reinforce the message * If properly supported by personal selling, it can be effective in changing behaviour	* Costly * Time consuming * Requires expertise in creating, updating data base and in developing and executing strategies
7.	Events Marketing	* Good at creating mass involvement and enthusiasm * Effective in getting corporate sponsorship * Provides good visibility	* Costly * Requires planning and logistics management expertise

The basic decision about what to say depends on the target audience, the benefits sought by the target audience, and the meaning and affect associated with different words and symbols, as perceived by the target segment. Taking all this into account, a health educator communicating the need for providing water to a child suffering from diarrhoea draws analogy with a leaking pitcher. A bureaucrat pours water over his bald head to explain the benefits of environmental conservation, the complexity of polio-drops and triple antigen gets simplified in 'Sishu Suraksha' (child protection) and so on.

Lessons to be learnt from these various success stories can be summarised as follows:

- Know your audience.
- Know the meanings associated with various words and symbols used by the target audience.
- Know the communication context (some words or symbols have different meanings and impact in different contexts in the same culture).
- Use social market research for the above and for testing the likely response.
- Keep it simple.
- Relate to the deeper sensibilities of people.

Messages need to be tested on the following :

- Are they believable?
- Are they promising a benefit important to the audience?
- Are they promising a unique benefit?
- Are they perceived to be different from others?

5.4.2   How should We Say it?

There is a debate amongst communication experts whether 'what to say' is more important than 'how to say it' for communication effectiveness. However, we hold the view that 'what you say' is more important than 'how you say it'. Nevertheless, 'how you say it' is of course also important. More so, in the context of complex developing world cultures with low literacy rates.

Some of the issues that must be considered in this regard are:

Rational vs. Emotional Appeal

Social marketing is mainly in the emotional domain but it is not devoid of rationality. Blood donors will not donate blood simply because somebody is dying if they are not reassured about the safety, hygiene and quick regeneration of blood (rational appeal). Mothers will not take their children to health camps simply out of affection or love, if some logical reason is not provided for it. Also, for getting attention, emotional appeals may work better in certain cultures but rational appeals may help with comprehension and conviction. Again, an emotional appeal at the right time and in a facilitative context may result in quick action or performance of desired behaviour.

Different Kinds of Emotional Appeals

Fear Appeal has to be within a threshold limit. If it is below a minimum threshold, it has no impact. If it crosses a higher limit, people ignore it in the absence of any coping mechanism. For example, the warning printed on cigarette packs 'Cigarette smoking is injurious to health', in many cultures, may be below the threshold level of causing concern, while another message showing a man turning into a skeleton when smoking a cigarette may be above the threshold of acceptance, and as a result gets ignored by hard core smokers. The impact may also differ across potential smokers, occasional smokers and hard core smokers. Experience in the context of family planning and mother and child welfare issues in the Indian context suggests that positive messages were found to be more effective than negative messages.

Humour Appeal attracts attention but distracts from comprehending the message. But different cultures have their own way of appreciating humour. Subtle humour may get the message across in some cultures. In other cultures it may not be noticed or understood. Humour has been used effectively in social messages in family planning, anti-alcohol consumption, literacy, mother and child welfare and so on. Most cultures also have very effective traditions of **satires**. These communicate the message without hurting anybody. Comprehension becomes easier. However, their impact on behavioural changes may or may not be there.

One Sided vs. Two Sided Messages

With a captive audience, having no preconceived notions, one sided messages are more effective. But with more knowledgeable or educated audiences putting across both pros and cons of an approach works better. For audiences with opposite views, it makes sense to begin with an agreement and then proceed with the contrary arguments.

Whether or not to Draw Conclusions

With captive, less educated audiences, it makes sense to draw conclusions. However, with educated audiences, it is better left to the audience.

Tone and Manner

This is extremely important for CASM communications, contextual relevance of different tones and manners need to be pre-tested.

Use of Analogies, Folklore, Phrases, Symbols and Mythological Characters

These are extremely important and effective in the CASM communication process. However, extreme care is required in understanding the subtle meanings. A slight change in words, may change meanings completely. Important symbols like the 'red cross (+)' have a universal appeal. The 'inverted red triangle' is recognised all over India as a symbol for family welfare. In the use of mythological characters, the religious sensitivity of the people has to be kept in mind.

Legal and Ethical Issues

As CASM often deals with socially sensitive issues, the legal and ethical aspects require a high level of attention.

To sum up, an effective message delivered in an interesting manner has better chances of achieving objectives than otherwise.

5.5 DECISIONS ON THE MEDIA AND ITS SCHEDULE

5.5.1 What are the Media Options Available for CASM?

CASM planners have plenty of media choices before them. In the broadest category they can choose from:

(A) **Mass-Media**
   * Print.
   * Audio.
   * Visual.
   * Audio-visual.
   * Posters and hoardings.
   * Transfers (mobile media like buses, trains and taxis).
   * Folk theatres, puppetry and other local media.

(B) **Interpersonal Media**
   * Direct Mail.
   * Telemarketing.
   * Personal presentation.

5.5.2 How do We Select which one or which Combination to Use?

The choice of media depends on the nature of the target audience and its media habits, communications objective, the task involved in terms of message and its execution, the cost and the availability of the media. Different media options or their combinations are also evaluated on the following three criteria (apart from those specified above):

- Outreach to the target audience.
- Frequency of exposure of target audience.
- Impact (credibility of the media with the target audience).
- Its cost.

Within each of the broad media options there are specific choices available. Print media consists of newspapers, magazines, hand-bills, newsletters, bulletins and so on. For social messages, which deal with deeper issues, short films, audio-visual programmes, local media like puppetry, theatre and street dramas have tremendous impact. Wall paintings have proved to be a cost-effective medium for creating awareness in rural areas. Television is a very powerful medium for effective social communication provided that the programmes are developed using a CASM approach.

A rural health agency in India learnt after some experimentation and after considerable time and expenditure that middle-aged local female workers accept mother and child welfare activities more easily than trained and professionally qualified nurses. Similarly, many political and socio-religious parties have very effectively combined mass-media and the support of local opinion leaders to create an impact. Understanding the social context in which the communication takes place or is hindered is extremely important for social communicators. Also, interpersonal channels are very important in generating action. Telemarketing has only a limited scope in many developing countries with low telephone density and cultural resistance towards talking to strangers on intimate issues. Some successes have been scored for telemarketing by Alcoholics Anonymous and certain social counselling agencies, where customers do not want to reveal their identity unless they develop trust in the counsellor or the counselling agency.

5.5.3 How Frequently should We Use Different Media?

Media scheduling is another important issue. People need to be continuously reminded, otherwise they forget. Some researchers suggest a minimum of three-exposures for a message to have some impact. Other researchers have suggested upto 6 exposures for a message to become part of long-term memory. There is also a question of seasonality. Certain actions have seasonal occurrences. People usually donate to charities when they get some discretionary income or during the festival season. For media planning and scheduling, professional help is a must. Many large agencies provide these services free of charge for good causes and many professional freelancers are available at reasonable rates.

5.6   DECISIONS ON THE MEDIA BUDGET

5.6.1   How do We Decide how much is Adequate?

The communication budget should be decided using the same principles as for the CASM budget (see 2.7). CASM communicators should keep in mind that high budgets do not necessarily mean more effectiveness and vice versa. Through creative integration, cost-effectiveness can be substantially improved. Also, many local innovative media, inspite of limited reach, have tremendous impact.

   The communication budget should be well planned; part of it should be treated as an investment for the future. It should never be treated as a discretionary expense to be increased or decreased depending on the availability of funds.

5.7   MONITORING AND EVALUATING CASM COMMUNICATION/PROMOTION ACTIVITIES

5.7.1   What and How do We Monitor and Evaluate?

CASM communication activities need to be periodically monitored and systematically evaluated using culturally-adapted social market research (CASOMAR). Messages need to be pre-tested (before they are released to the media) and post-tested (to test the impact after the release). Media effectiveness needs to be evaluated. The key factors in evaluation are:

- Clarity of objectives.
- Cultural sensitivity of methodology.
- In-depth understanding of the target groups.

5.7.2 How can We Continue Improving the Effectiveness of Our Communication/Promotion?

CASM planners need to keep the following aspects in mind for continuously improving their effectiveness and efficiency:

- Know your audience through CASOMAR and regular interaction.
- Both short- and long-term communication objectives must be clearly defined.
- The communication-mix and the balancing of 'pull versus push' must be carefully worked out.
- Importance, credibility and uniqueness of the message must be ensured.
- Impact must be ensured by means of symbols and attention to details in execution.
- Appropriate media-mix and scheduling, objectives, audiences' media habits and the message requirement must always be kept in mind. (For example, for complex demonstrations on personal hygiene, audio-visual aids are more effective than audio or even print media).
- An adequate budget must be prepared.
- The importance of messages by word of mouth must be recognised.
- An adequate CASOMAR arrangement must be in place to plan, execute, monitor and evaluate the CASM activities. Wherever organisational capabilities are inadequate, CASM organisations can network effectively to augment or supplement their resources.

To sum up, we would like to highlight what the main factors making for an effective CASM communication are:

i) **Knowing the target audience through CASOMAR and regular interactions.**
ii) **Knowing one's own objectives and capabilities.**
iii) **Keeping it simple.**
iv) **Using a professional approach.**
v) **Continuously using CASOMAR for monitoring and evaluation.**

5.8   RECOMMENDED READING

Bird, Drayton (1989). *Commonsense Direct Marketing*, Kogan Page, London.

Ogilvy, D. (1983). *Ogilvy on Advertising*, Pan Books, London.

Rothschild, M.L. (1979). 'Marketing Communications in Non-Business Situations or Why It's So Hard to Sell Brotherhood Like Soap' *Journal of Marketing*, 43, Spring , pp. 11–20.

Strenthal, B. and **C.S. Craig** (December 1974). 'Fear Appeals, Revisited and Revised', *Journal of Consumer Research*, 3, pp. 23–34.

Chapter 6

Management of CASM Activities

Mithileshwar Jha

CASM activities need to be carefully managed. The relevant activities and critical issues involved are outlined in Table 6.1.

Table 6.1
CASM Managerial Activities and Major Issues

Serial Number	Activity	Major Issues
1	Analysis and planning	1.1 How do we review and analyse our present situation? 1.2 What do we plan to achieve? 1.3 How do we achieve it?
2	Organising	2.1 What are the tasks to be performed? 2.2 What kind of competence is required for the effective performance of the tasks? 2.3 How should different functionaries relate to each other? 2.4 How do we allocate resources?
3	Implementing	3.1 How do we select, train and retain competent personnel? 3.2 How do we ensure effective and efficient execution?
4	Review and facilitate	4.1 What do we review? 4.2 How do we review and facilitate better performance?

The major issues for each activity are discussed here:

6.1 OVERALL PLANNING AND ANALYSIS

6.1.1 How do We Review and Analyse Our Present Situation?

The key requirements for this are:

- A good data base. (This may require designing simple formats to generate relevant data, and a computer with basic software for entering, processing and retrieving data. Small NGOs can even maintain manual databases).

- Specific data generated through CASOMAR.
- Committed professionals with analytical minds and experience based insight. Such individuals may be hard to find but it is well worth it to search for people with these potentials.
- Involvement of all personnel in the planning process. The basic tasks are CASOMAR, situation analyses using SWOT and competence framework (see 2.2.1).

6.1.2   What do We Plan to Achieve?

This involves the following:

- *Defining Constituency and Scope of Activities*

  Each CASM organisation has a wide choice of constituencies (client universe) and scope of activities. The broad guideline for the choice can be as follows:

  * Define the broad constituencies of interest.
  * Identify the capabilities and interest of the organisation both current and future.
  * Shortlist the constituencies and activities using a matrix.

  Constituency attractiveness can be defined in terms of:

  * Meaningfulness of the constituency need.
  * Its size.
  * Its criticality of need.
  * Proximity.
  * Accessibility.
  * Actionability.

  CASM activities need to be prioritised keeping the important needs of the selected constituencies in mind. Even when CASM organisations begin with a preconceived set of activities, they soon adapt and get into other related and unrelated activities. However, CASM organisations should keep in mind the following:

  * **They must have focus.** They normally have limited resources. It should not be frittered away on too many things.
  * They should consider **networking** with other organisations and encourage voluntary efforts and people's initiative to supplement their activities. New activities should be carefully considered before being adopted.

- *Defining the Organisational Mission*

  It may be debated whether the mission should determine the constituency and activity-mix or whether it should be the other way around. Deciding on constituency with a broad idea about what the organisation is interested in and capable of and then refining it with a clear idea of the mission may be a desirable approach. A good mission statement should:

★ Pose a sufficient challenge.
★ Provide some superior goals.
★ Be distinctive and simple.
★ Provide broad guidelines for operation.

The overall mission should always be defined in a participatory manner. It should be discussed and accepted across the organisation. It should be communicated in a wide manner and activities should be periodically evaluated in the light of the broad mission statement.

- *Defining the Mission*

CASM organisations normally thrive on ambiguity. Ambiguity has its own benefits in terms of creative problem solving and developing intuitive insights. However, it is desirable that an organisation have some specific goals. While the mission provides the broad aims and aspirations, objectives help in concretising them into achievable, tangible factors. For example, an organisation dealing with child immunisation may have the following objectives:

(a) Short-term (the following year)

★ Increase awareness about the benefits of immunisation among young mothers in the target area from the current 30 per cent to 60 per cent.
★ Improve the knowledge of 30 per cent of the mothers who are aware of the importance of child hygiene.
★ Immunise 30 per cent of the children below the age of five.

(b) Long-term (two to three years)

★ Achieve awareness rates of more than 70 per cent.
★ Improve the knowledge of 60 per cent of mothers.
★ Immunise more than 60 per cent of the children below the age of five.
★ Develop an image of a friendly, caring organisation, providing quality service in a cost-effective manner.

The above objectives have the following features:

★ They elaborate on short-term and long-term aspects.
★ They cover both qualitative and quantitative aspects.
★ They have a specific time frame.

Specific objectives should not lead to target orientation. They should help in marshalling resources, fixing a time-frame and providing some clarity about what can be achieved and what is possible.

6.2   OPERATIONAL CONSIDERATIONS

6.2.1   What are the Tasks to be Performed?

In simple terms programme directors—who will also frequently be responsible for their organisation's CASM—are expected to perform the following spectrum of tasks:

- ★ Listen
- ★ Read
- ★ Communicate
  - Speak
  - Write
  - Make presentations
- ★ Mobilise
- ★ Facilitate
- ★ Motivate

- ★ Lead
- ★ Negotiate
- ★ Co-ordinate, conduct meetings
- ★ Analyse
- ★ Plan
- ★ Decide, act
- ★ Manage conflicts
- ★ Manage co-operation

6.2.2 What Kind of Competence is Required for the Effective Performance of these Tasks?

The requirements are grouped under three broad categories of knowledge, skill and attitude.

- **Knowledge:** Development professionals need to have a broad understanding of the following:
  - ★ Macro and micro economic factors.
  - ★ Socio-cultural norms and practices.
  - ★ Project management.
  - ★ Basic accounting and finance.
  - ★ Basic marketing and social marketing.
  - ★ Knowledge of self and client groups.
  - ★ Management of change.
  - ★ Donor agency norms.
  - ★ Development economics, administration and political processes.

- **Skill:** Development professionals need to possess at least some of the following abilities:
  - ★ People skills (relationship building, motivating).
  - ★ Planning skills.
  - ★ Analytical/problem solving skills.
  - ★ Social skills.
  - ★ Communication skills.
  - ★ Negotiation skills.
  - ★ Listening skills.
  - ★ Political skills and execution skills.

- **Attitude:** The desired features in a development professional are:
  - ★ Empathy (i.e., the ability to put oneself in the shoes of others).
  - ★ Humility.
  - ★ Sense of purpose.
  - ★ Responsiveness.
  - ★ Ownership of task.
  - ★ Perseverance.
  - ★ High degree of tolerance for ambiguity.

The requirements will vary across task situations. We have provided only an illustrative list here. Even then it is a tall order. Organisations recruiting or training personnel for a specific task may use this as a checklist and prioritise the items that may be more important in their context.

6.2.3   How would Different Functions Relate to Each Other?

In this context there are two important elements to consider:

- ### The Organisation Structure

    CASM organisations should be flat (with as few levels as possible), non-bureaucratic and non-hierarchical. They should be client-focused, adaptive and entrepreneurial. A flexible team-based approach for innovations and a geographical-cum-functional approach for routine/maintenance operations may be desirable (see Figure 6.1).

Figure 6.1
Functional Organisation

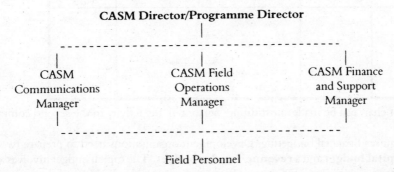

The basic organisation can be suitably adapted to focus on specific client groups (e.g., women or old people) or on specialised tasks, e.g., income generation versus health or education, specific groups or individuals. In smaller organisations one or two persons can perform all the tasks with or without the support of part-time employees and/or volunteers.

- ### The Systems

    For any organisation to function smoothly the systems mentioned above are necessary. These can be both formal and informal. They need to be simple, easily understood, user friendly, (for both organisation personnel and clients), they should facilitate improved performance and provide timely feedback. **One key feature of a CASM organisational structure and system should be to allow freedom and space for the personnel to give their best. Experimentation, tolerance for failure, open discussion, constructive dissent, questioning assumptions, learning and adapting while doing, should be promoted keeping client interest at the centre.** Needless to say, it requires a high degree of concern on the part of the organisation for its own personnel, both in terms of pay and other facilities. For smaller organisations, the co-ordination across functions and personnel could be achieved through frequent interactions—both formal and informal. In larger groups, committees with identified co-ordinators (who are rotated periodically) can serve this purpose. **Such committees exist to seek new, more and better ways of diagnosing issues and developing corrective actions in an action dominated mode.**

6.2.4   How do We Allocate Resources?

CASM organisational resources include time of the personnel, money, other tangible resources (like transport, facilities) and client groups' time and resources. For most development organisations, the most **critical** resource is **'personnel time'** and the most **scarce** resource is **money**. Allocating resources for various activities in the short- and long-term period is a key and regular managerial activity.

For allocating personnel time, a simple approach could be to develop a chart as shown in Figure 6.2.

Figure 6.2
Activity and Manpower Resource Scheduling

Sl. No.	Activity (prioritised)	Time sequence (days/weeks/months)	Individuals responsible
1			
2		- - - - - - - - - -	
3		- - - - - - - - - -	
		- - - - - - - - - -	

(*Note*: A similar chart can be made substituting 'personnel' for activity in the second column)

Allocating money requires financial budgeting. Development organisations need to prepare two kinds of budgets, namely, a **capital budget** and a **revenue/regular budget.** The capital budget involves allocation of resources for **assets** (e.g., buildings, furniture, office equipment and vehicles) and the revenue budget deals with regular incomes and expenses. Some caveats for the allocation of financial resources are:

i)   One should take a long-term view (e.g., buying an obsolete computer can save money today, but can prove to be costly in the long run in terms of maintenance and incompatibility with new software).

ii)   Investments in *softer* things like various low-cost software, consulting help, etc. need careful consideration. What may look to be wasteful or low priority to begin with may yield substantial savings and return in the long run.

iii)   Complementarity in investments should be kept in mind. Buying computer hardware without provision for the essential software and training of personnel may yield only a high-tech look.

iv)   Development organisations need to invest in making their working environment decent (not luxurious) with well located offices, functional layouts, comfortable furniture and other basic facilities.

The allocation of resources must be done in a consultative process and in a transparent manner.

6.3   IMPLEMENTATION

6.3.1   How do We Select and Train Competent Personnel?

CASM organisations should first develop appropriate job specifications and then decide on the education required for key jobs (see 6.2.1 and 6.2.2). Selection could be through personal contacts, announcing jobs in select institutions and places, releasing formal advertisements followed by interviews, etc. The key issue is reaching and attracting talents with the right attitudes. Some key factors in this regard are the image of the organisation and its leader, the nature of the job, the challenges and the way these are communicated, the working environment, the pay and perks, and future prospect.

6.3.2   How do We Retain Efficient Personnel?

For retaining personnel, the determining variables are the organisational culture, facilitative leadership, freedom to perform, fair and decent renumeration and responsive client groups.

The critical requirements in this context are:

- Putting the right person on the right job.
- Encouraging the staff to participate in decision-making.
- Consultative planning (involving the field staff) to develop a sufficient understanding of the basic objectives among the field personnel. It should facilitate two things:

    a)   Relating to the **'big picture'** (higher level goals) even while doing mundane things.
    b)   **Local adaptation** without compromising the main objectives.

- Role clarity among the field personnel to avoid confusion but with sufficient scope for individual initiative.
- Simple, fast, formal and informal communication channels.
- Facilitative leadership.
- Community participation at every stage.
- A bias for action and action-oriented learning.

6.4   REVIEW AND FACILITATION

6.4.1   What do We Review?

The purpose of review is to facilitate better performance rather than control individuals or resources. Development organisations need to review the following periodically:

- Client satisfaction and involvement (quarterly or half yearly).

- Achievements compared with goals/objectives (for diagnosing reasons for shortfalls or excesses) (quarterly).
- Utilisation of resources (quarterly with a view to improving resource allocation and utilisation).
- Satisfaction of the organisation's personnel (annually).

6.4.2   How do We Review and Facilitate Better Performance?

CASM review systems should be simple, user-friendly, facilitative rather than control oriented, continuous and flexible. The focus should be on learning, improving and involving/motivating all concerned.

In the long run (every three to five years), CASM projects/programmes should be assessed/evaluated for their impact in terms of achievement of long-term objectives by conducting a comprehensive **social audit**. CASOMAR can be of immense help in this.

To sum up, development organisations should appreciate a three stage programme learning curve:

- Stage 1: Learning to be effective
- Stage 2: Learning to be efficient
- Stage 3: Learning to expand.

Effective CASM management requires:

- Focus on specific client groups, and on specific areas of organisational competence.
- Personnel who are competent, compassionate, courageous and committed to the cause.
- A facilitative leadership.
- Simple, meaningful, personalised communication systems.
- A vibrant, learning-oriented organisational ethos.
- Demanding, yet partnership-oriented, client groups including donors and facilitators.
- Emphasis on efficient use of all resources, subject to first achieving effectiveness norms.

The satisfaction of having made some difference in society is the real reward for development/CASM managers. The question is not whether these tasks should be performed, but whether we can do them better and with more efficient use of resources.

6.5   HOW TO DRAW UP A MODEL CASM PLAN

A model step-by-step development of a CASM plan framework is set out in Table 6.2.

Table 6.2
A Model CASM Plan Framework

Steps		Issues/Questions	Refer Section
1. CASOMAR	1.1	Who should be targeted?	3.1
	1.2	How does the target audience perceive the project objectives?	3.2.2
2. Cultural-adaptation	2.1	Project-specific KCVs	4.2.1
3. Situation analysis	3.1	What are the opportunities and threats offered by the environment?	2.2.1
	3.2	What are the needs of the client group?	2.2.1
	3.3	What capabilities (strength, weakness) we have to respond to the opportunities and threats?	2.2.1
4. Setting objectives	4.1	What should be the short-term objectives?	2.2.2
	4.2	What should be the long-term objectives?	2.2.2
5. Broad strategy for achieving the objectives	5.1	Who should be the target client group?	2.2.3 'A'
	5.2	What should be the image/relationship and broad approach vis-à-vis different client groups?	2.2.3 'B'
6. CASM-mix	6.1	What should be the 8Ps of the CASM-mix	2.3
7. CASM budget	7.1	What should be the CASM budget?	2.7
8. CASM review and facilitation	8.1	What should be reviewed?	2.8 and 6.4
	8.2	How can performance be improved?	

6.6 RECOMMENDED READING

Drucker, P.F. (1986–1991). *Innovation and Entrepreneurship: Practice and Principles*, East–West Press, New Delhi.
——— (1990). *Managing the Non-Profit Organisation: Principles and Practices*, Butterworth-Heinemann, Oxford.

Kasturirangan, V., S. Karim and **S.K. Sandberg** (1996). 'Do Better at Doing Good', *Harvard Business Review*, May–June, pp. 42–54.

Korten, D.C. (1981). 'Social Development: Putting People First', in D.C. Korten and F.B. Alfonso (eds), *Bureaucracy and the Poor: Closing the Gap*, McGraw-Hill, pp. 214–16.

Payne, A.F. (1988). 'Developing a Marketing Oriented Organization' *Business Horizons*, May–June, pp. 46–53.

Slater, S.F. and **J.C. Narver** (1995). 'Market Orientation and the Learning Organization', *Journal of Marketing*, 59, pp. 63–74.

Waterman, Jr., R.H., T.J. Peters and **J.R. Phillips** (1980). 'Structure is Not Organization', *Business Horizons*, June, pp. 14–26.

Ziethmal, V.A., A. Parasuraman and **L.L. Berry** (1990). *Delivering Quality Service*, The Free Press, New York.

Part III

Some CASM Case Studies

Case Study A

Safe Motherhood Approaches Using Culturally-appropriate Methods in the Highlands of Papua New Guinea and Other Examples

Marie-Therese Feuerstein

 A.1 INTRODUCTION

This case study refers to an integrated rural development project in a highland province of Papua New Guinea (PNG). For the past three years culturally-appropriate approaches have been employed to contact communities, elicit their interest in co-operative action, and enable them to articulate and prioritise their development needs. The project (agriculture, marketing, health, education and women's development) has responded by tailoring its inputs and activities around such needs. The case study focuses on how the complex and previously taboo issues of human sexuality and safe motherhood have been raised and how practical and culturally-appropriate approaches and actions have been identified and begun to be implemented. The concluding part of this case study outlines some examples of culturally-appropriate social marketing which have been used elsewhere in the world, in the context of safe motherhood, family planning and reproductive health.

A.2 THE COMPLEX SOCIO-CULTURAL CONTEXT OF HIGHLAND PAPUA NEW GUINEA

After its first contact with Europeans in the 16th century, PNG was at the end of the last century divided between the Dutch, British and Germans. After the First World War Australia captured the German section. During the Second World War much of the island was captured by the Japanese. Then, after the war, it was liberated and administered by Australia. In 1975, PNG became an independent country within the Commonwealth. Its population was reported to be over four million in 1995. Strictly speaking, PNG is not a 'poor' country; its per capita GNP was US $1120 in 1995. The illiteracy level is reported to be 65 per cent for females and 55 per cent for males, and life expectancy is 54 years. There are 19 provinces, and the country has been 'decentralised' since the 1980s. Today, cultural differences are still extraordinarily high, despite a growing homogenisation of behaviour and ideology under the strong influences generated by the forces of the church, the state and the cash economy.

The integrated rural development project is located in the highland province of Simbu. The pre-modern history of PNG remains largely unknown, as there are no written accounts. It was widely believed that the highland region was uninhabited. Then, in the 1930s, explorers, traders and missionaries ventured into the highlands. They discovered that the region was heavily populated, having probably been settled ten thousand years ago. The fertile highland valleys attested to the agricultural skills of the inhabitants. In fact, they were probably among the world's first settled farmers. The people at first cordially greeted the outsiders, but it was the latter who fired the first shots which produced fatalities. The next group of visitors were greeted with hostility. The highlanders at first thought that the pale-faced outsiders were spirits of their dead ancestors. They did not know about or use metal, animal power, or the wheel, and used shells as 'money'. Individual ownership was considered second to communal ownership. There was an in-built 'social security' system. Ceremonial exchanges of surplus wealth (e.g., pigs) took place as a sign of prestige and to obligate receivers. Prowess in battle was valued in the warrior society. Clan loyalties were fierce.

Today, the 26,400 Simbus live in family, clan and tribal groupings. The pre-1930s society was in itself fragmented by the clan and tribal system. There are still reported to be many different languages spoken in PNG. The steep mountainous terrain leaves insufficient arable land. The small provincial capital, straddling the poorly maintained Highlands highway, houses government offices, a hospital, churches, and the project headquarters. Levels of out-migration are high. Two of the seven districts are very remote, one with access only by air. There is no large-scale agriculture, wage employment is insufficient, and most incomes are regarded as being 'below the poverty level'. There is considerable popular dissatisfaction, and social unrest has spilled over into the turbulent urban areas of towns and PNG's capital. The provincial government has recently banned alcohol in the province.

A.3 AN INTEGRATED RURAL DEVELOPMENT PROJECT

This five-year project conducted in five districts aims to increase economic activity, household income and welfare in north Simbu through self-sustaining local initiatives and decentralised district level planning and decision-making. This is to be done by promoting the work of government extension services that give support for community self-reliance and by fostering participation by the government in the planning and development of activities sponsored by the community. In addition, the project aims to enhance food security as well as income earning opportunities through adequate technical support services provided by government, promotion of smallholder development of particular cash-earning enterprises, and improvement of rural access in the more remote parts of the province through a programme of road-building and maintenance. Finally, the project aims to improve health, nutrition and education levels in the community. Health activities include strengthening of the 'cold chain' (which necessitates cooler equipment to retain the low temperatures necessary to preserve vaccines), upgrading health infrastructure, equipping mobile health patrols, establishing two-way radio contact between the hospital and isolated health centres, increasing the availability of safe water and sanitation, helping the population to protect itself better from malaria, and establishing in-service training for health workers.

A.4 THE HEALTH CONTEXT WHICH SPEARHEADED ACTION FOR SAFE MOTHERHOOD

A.4.1 The State of General Health

A 1994 participatory exercise (which was multidisciplinary and involved provincial health officials, project staff, representatives of district staff, health adviser/facilitator) to plan the health component of the project, revealed that common diseases and conditions causing death and disability were diarrhoeal diseases (principally due to unclean food preparation and feeding practices), upper respiratory infections (particularly among children), preventable childhood diseases (like measles, polio, whooping cough, tetanus,), tuberculosis and malaria. There was also found to be a high incidence of death and disability among child-bearing women and their new-born infants.

A.4.2 The State of Women's Health

A report on the state of women's health in PNG claimed that maternal mortality in PNG, defined as non-accidental deaths during pregnancy or within 42 days of termination of pregnancy, reaches levels of 120 per 10,000 live births. Around 60 per cent of births were not supervised by trained personnel. There was a high proportion of infection in new-born children due to untreated sexually transmitted diseases in the mothers. Although fertility was rising, net reproduction rate was estimated to be about 2.3 per cent. A 1994 study found that some of the risk factors causing such mortality and disability did not rest with the people themselves, but with the health care services available to them. For example, an inadequately funded, inadequately staffed and inadequately trained health service promotes numerous risk factors to the population at large. These issues cannot generally be addressed at the community level, but must be taken up by the authorities vested with responsibility for these functions.

A.5 THE FRAGILE NETWORK OF HEALTH SERVICES

In Simbu province there is a new, Japanese built, 200-bed provincial hospital, district health centres (one is like a small district hospital run by the Catholic Church), sub-health centres, and aid posts (serving around 5000 people)—often constructed by local communities from 'bush materials'. There are also mobile maternal and child health (MCH) patrols.

A.5.1 Shortage of Funds

Various interlinked problems were found, in 1994, to be hindering the achievement of maternal and child health goals. Multiple layers of unco-ordinated management and decision-making complicated the provision of streamlined support to districts and effective responses to community needs. The 'cold chain' weakened by lack of cooler equipment hindered effective immunisation coverage. The isolation of some communities in the mountainous province prevented easy access to health services, especially in obstetric and other emergencies. The health service system was struggling under the burden of lack of financial and other resources. Funds to replace or repair anything from burnt-down aid posts to medical equipment were scarce. Transportation was not easily available for district staff. MCH patrols, once the pride of PNG (which trekked for 1–5 days, climbing and carrying clinic equipment and medicines) were frequently cancelled due to tribal fighting. There were few 'camping allowances' to cover staff expenses. Health staff were even forced to flee from aid posts or health centres during tribal clashes. Even where communities did build aid posts, funds were not always available to station a health worker there. Most health posts had water and electricity problems. Sometimes water was diverted upstream by disputing tribes during tribal clashes, or siphoned off from the plastic piping.

A.5.2   Shortage of Equipment

In the maternity units at health centres, some health staff did not even have a blood pressure machine, or simple suction methods for extracting mucous from the mouth/nose of the new-born. In at least one centre, staff re-used disposable gloves, and lighting was so inadequate that they sometimes had to light old cardboard to be able to see at crucial times in the labour ward. There was also a scarcity of treatment recording forms. Some staff were using the backs of schoolbook pages or old calendars to record patient information and the results of school health checks. Staff often felt demoralised, and let standards of practice drop.

A.6   FINDING CULTURALLY-APPROPRIATE APPROACHES TO SAFE MOTHERHOOD AND NEW-BORN CARE

A.6.1   An Exploratory Workshop

An exploratory workshop was held in the provincial capital of Kundiawa in May 1995. It was attended by 32 participants, including health staff in charge of district health centres, district women's development officers, representatives of women organisations, literacy activists, church health services, and Kundiawa hospital staff. Village women had particularly expressed the need to learn more about 'hygienic village deliveries', and to have someone in their own village trained to conduct safe and clean childbirth. The workshop was a first step in assessing the local situation and preparing for action. There were two types of culture, the rich but problematic local popular context, and the culture of deprivation currently prevailing in the health service system. In order to initiate work with the communities it was first necessary to examine and where possible strengthen the health services to enable them to do this. Meanwhile community contacts continued to be made by the non-health components of the project as they mobilised interested communities to analyse their situation and prioritise their various development needs. The challenge for the health component of the project was to develop a two-pronged strategy culturally-appropriate to both communities and health service.

A.6.2   A Revolving Fund

One culturally-appropriate response was activated when during the Safe Motherhood workshop a Revolving Fund for Instruments and Equipment was officially launched. The idea was to give priority to instrument and equipment needs of health staff and voluntary workers in remote locations, where there were high rates of maternal and new-born mortality and disability. The fund is administered by local senior nurses, and has a local bank account. The revolving fund system is not a commercially oriented system. The consumer takes full responsibility for the purchase of items from a selection of 11 priority instruments and equipment, and receives instructions on how best to take care of the items. Items can be paid for over several months. A subsidy scheme is underway for more expensive items. This scheme is also designed to facilitate the local purchase of equipment available in trade stores (such as kerosene lamps, batteries, plastic sheeting, buckets, razor blades and hold-alls) which are needed by the existing and the newly trained traditional birth attendants (TBAs).

A.6.3   Emphasis on Mother-friendliness

Another culturally-appropriate response, resulting from analysis of reluctance by local women to deliver in health centres/aid posts, was the development of a simple 'Checklist: Are You Mother-friendly?' (see Chart A. 1). This helped health staff identify what needed to be done to make their services more culturally-appropriate. Plans were made to train more traditional birth attendants, as attempts had been positive in an earlier project area in the southern part of the province, where, despite sparse support or supervision, TBAs continued to assist women by providing clean birth techniques. Another challenging area in which culturally-appropriate responses needed to be found was that of family planning.

A.7   FAMILY PLANNING APPROACHES TARGETED AT MEN

A.7.1   Low Family Planning Coverage

In 1994, the project drew attention to the fact that in the Simbu province less than 2 per cent of couples in their reproductive age were estimated to be using any form of family planning. Existing family planning methods were primarily female methods, and were integrated with MCH services. This did not match the interest in, and needs for, family planning by men. Strategies were suggested to increase male acceptance of family planning, including community-based contraceptive distribution tailored to cultural customs and preferences.

Chart A.1

Are You Mother-friendly?

A Checklist for Assessment

Many women prefer to have their babies at home because hospital health centres may seem unfriendly. These questions can help to assess whether there is a truly mother-friendly atmosphere at hospital/health centre/aid post. They are intended to supplement existing criteria for a baby-friendly hospital.

Antenatal Care

- ☐ Is antenatal check up, including tetanus immunisation, available everyday and is iron/foliate given to pregnant women?
- ☐ Is information on early recognition of complications prominently displayed and communicated to each woman?
- ☐ Do staff avoid unfriendly or judgmental attitudes when dealing with women, especially in cases of abortion complications?
- ☐ Are staff welcoming and friendly to those accompanying the women, whether TBA or family?
- ☐ Do staff explain procedures to the women and her family?

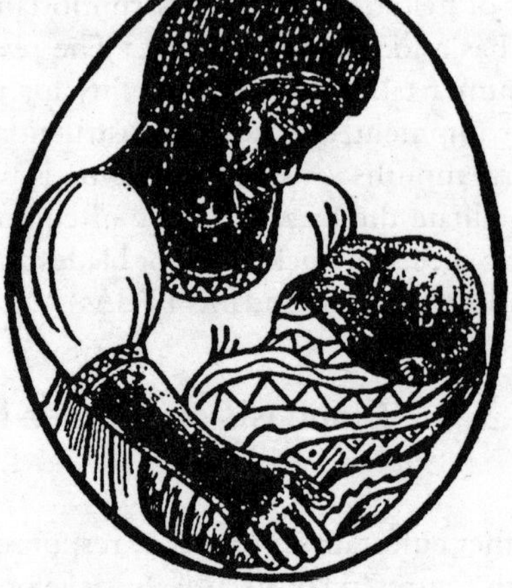

Delivery Care

- ☐ Are husbands, partners or other persons accompanying the woman encouraged to remain with her during labour if she would like it?
- ☐ Are care providers polite and considerate?
- ☐ Do staff set aside time to explain the process of labour and delivery?
- ☐ Do staff listen and respond to women's concerns?
- ☐ Are unnecessary medical routines/interventions avoided (e.g., espisiotomy, shaving, enemas)?
- ☐ Are flexible routines followed during labour and in choice of birthing position?
- ☐ Are traditional practices that are not harmful respected and encouraged?
- ☐ May women have privacy if they wish?
- ☐ Are strict standards of clean delivery maintained?
- ☐ Is immediate mother-baby skin contact encouraged and is the baby breast-fed as soon as the mother is ready?

Post-partum Care

- ☐ Are babies kept in close contact with mothers and is feeding on demand encouraged?
- ☐ Are mothers and families advised about nutrition and rest after delivery?
- ☐ Is appropriate new-born care available, including resuscitation?
- ☐ Are families encouraged to visit and celebrate the birth of the baby?
- ☐ Are mothers given health education and advice on leaving hospital/health centre?

Contraception Services

- ☐ Is counselling provided to all women who have had an abortion before leaving hospital?
- ☐ Are family planning information and services available to all mothers on all days?
- ☐ Are such information and services provided to men (by a male care provider, if necessary)?

Emergency Care

- ☐ Is immediate attention/priority given to emergencies?
- ☐ Are steps for admission welcoming, simple and rapid?
- ☐ Are facilities available round the clock for surgery and blood transfusion?
- ☐ Are medications and operative interventions used in accordance with recommended norms/indicators?
- ☐ Are all maternal deaths audited and reported?

A.7.2   Family Planning Targeting

In most countries, men have seldom been asked what they know and do about family planning. It is often assumed that they have little interest. But, men need to be recognised as important and interested participants in family planning. They need to be encouraged to think about family size and child-spacing. Men become interested in family planning principally for the sake of their children's welfare, and also for that of their wives. Studies indicate that although men are willing to share responsibility for family planning decisions, many still prefer that the woman take responsibility for actually using the contraceptive method. Sometimes men themselves have conflicting views within themselves about family planning. For example, while regarding small families as being good in principle, they continue to have more respect for women with large families. They continue to divorce women who cannot bear children.

A.7.3   Fertility Surveys

Most fertility studies in the past have focused on women. The few surveys that targeted men found that while men favour family planning, they still think that it might undermine their authority as head of the family. Others oppose it on religious grounds, or fear what they regard as harmful side effects of using contraceptives. Others desire children as a sign of virility, and to enhance their prestige in the community. In Simbu province, an important cultural variable is the need for male offspring in relation to retaining power for tribal fights. Most couples still believe in the importance of having male children to retain clan power and security.

A.7.4   Factors Influencing Sexual Behaviour

Traditional customs called for separate houses for men and women; pre-marital sex and adultery were not tolerated; a breast-feeding woman had to abstain from marital relations until her child was weaned. Such customary patterns have been eroded by 'modernisation' and urbanisation. Marriage patterns may now result in couples spending much more time in each other's company, thus necessitating even more the need for family planning and child-spacing. Polygamous living patterns also necessitate the use of family planning, and are particularly prone to dangers of HIV/AIDS/STD transmission.

A.7.5   Lack of Family Planning Information

Studies elsewhere indicate that lack of appropriate and accessible information on family planning rather than opposition to it is a main reason given for men not using family planning. Lack of communication between husband and wife is another reason. In Simbu culture, it is still not common for parents to discuss human sexuality and family planning with their children. Where human sexuality and family planning are taught in school under 'biology', teachers are often uncomfortable teaching these subjects. Only girls, not boys, are taught about family planning in school. There is an increasing problem of unplanned teenage pregnancies in the province. However, the 1994 study indicated that Papua New Guineans are generally quite capable of discussing sexual matters when the issues are important, when their privacy is protected, and when they trust the interviewer. Generally, few health workers make an effort to explain the nature of disease or treatment to their patients. Others know too little or are too uncertain of what they know to attempt health education. Improving the capacity for sexual health education within the health services should be a high priority, requiring new positions and specialised training. Urban life and changing social values influence decisions about family size. For example, due to urbanisation there is often a greater desire to educate the children, provide medical care, and better economic opportunities.

A.7.6   Male Dominance

In Simbu, a wife is usually economically dependent on her husband, although it is she who produces the food crops, takes care of the household, children and livestock. There is evidence that disposable cash income is often squandered by men on beer and gambling. Disposable income is also used to purchase tinned food from trade stores.

Men usually learn about contraception in Simbu from their wives, friends or the mass media, but seldom from health care providers. A common fear among men is that a wife using contraceptives may be unfaithful. Men need easily accessible, high quality services, and encouragement to support their wife's use of contraceptives. Studies elsewhere have found that the attitude of the husband was the reason which women gave most often for not using family planning methods. Although most men often know something about family planning, knowledge of specific contraceptive methods is often limited. Sometimes men know more about female than male contraceptive methods. They need to know where to get services and supplies for men, such as condoms or vasectomy. In Simbu province there are also religious cultural variables to consider. For example, Catholics prefer 'natural' family planning.

A.7.7   Male Ignorance

In Simbu, the key questions identified by men were: What do men actually know about family planning; do they know where to obtain services; what are their attitudes towards family planning; what messages will appeal to men; what media will reach them; what information and services do men want; how do they want services and supplies delivered; what services are already available for men; are those services well publicised; are they affordable to men; are those services being used by men; how can those services be improved? **A small-scale survey was suggested to obtain this information. Another method could be to conduct focus group discussions**.

A.7.8   Social Marketing of Family Planning

From experience elsewhere in the world, twelve principles have been identified for designing family planning services for men. These are:

- Services and products must be well publicised, for example through magazines, newspapers, radio, TV, posters, and literacy materials.
- The publicity and messages must be tailored to men's needs and aspirations, making them active participants. For example, messages can emphasise how men can benefit from family planning, and how it can enhance their esteem. Messages can appeal to men's sense of responsibility to support their family. Topics of special interest, like sports, card-playing, (or in the case of Simbu dart-playing) can be used for promoting family planning.
- Training men to counsel other men can provide a sympathetic source of information and advice. For example, family planning associations in Indonesia have used male counsellors successfully. Young males can be trained to work with youth.
- Satisfied consumers can be enlisted to promote male-oriented methods, and to counsel other men. This is particularly important for vasectomy, about which men often have wrong information and apprehensions. Most men who have had vasectomies did so only after talking to other men who had a vasectomy; also, clinic staff and outreach workers who have had vasectomies have proved useful in counselling other men about vasectomy.
- Health staff, counsellors and administrative personnel can also be trained to encourage men's participation in family planning. They need to understand what information, advice and services men want, and to promote male-oriented family planning methods.
- Where resources allow, separate family planning clinics for men can be useful. They could offer comprehensive reproductive health services, including diagnosis and treatment of infertility and sexually transmitted diseases.
- Clinics which serve both men and women should be hospitable to men, with leaflets and posters designed to interest men as well as women. Setting aside some clinic hours each week just for men may also improve male attendance at clinics.
- Like all other family planning services, special services for men should respect individual privacy.
- Men must be able to obtain the services they want when they need them. More men can be served if more methods such as condoms, natural family planning and vasectomy are made available to them. If instruction in particular methods are not available, men should be referred to where they can obtain such services.
- Services should be readily available at community and workplace levels. For example, condoms can be made available at places like bars, stores, hairdressers, as well as clinics. Community-based contraceptive distributors are used in various countries to increase availability and use by men.
- Services should be available at times convenient for men, usually outside working hours. In Thailand, one hospital began vasectomy clinics during the weekends, and saw a rise in clients.
- Men should be encouraged, as far as possible, to be present when their wives/partners give birth. Many men are not really aware of the process of labour. It has been found that when they are aware, they are more interested in family planning. An important time to offer information and advice to couples is the immediate period after a birth.

As far as Simbu province is concerned, the suggestions from men, particularly those involved in literacy activities, were as follows:

- Special clinics to be held at the village level to inform and motivate both men and women to use family planning;

- Community dialogue to discuss patterns of sexual behaviour and family planning using locally produced visual aids and learning approaches such as posters, charts, drama, songs, and a locally produced video, designed and produced with adolescent participation;
- A daily, serialised, soap opera-style radio programme designed to encourage men's participation in family planning;
- A hospital-based clinic/drop-in centre with full-time staff to deal with male family planning clients, and also HIV/AIDS/STDs and infertility;
- An adolescent health programme designed for high schools and vocational schools to tackle the subjects of sexual health, HIV/AIDS/STDs and family planning, and stressing positive family life values and behaviour;
- Literacy teachers trained to increase awareness of family planning and reproductive health;
- A survey of community attitudes concerning men and family planning in selected rural and urban areas;
- District awareness groups to co-ordinate and monitor local activities (mobile units composed of government officials, NGO representatives, and community-based organisations); awareness raising during village and district women's group meetings.

A.8 CULTURALLY-APPROPRIATE SOCIAL MARKETING TO MOBILISE COMMUNITIES

'Selling' a community development, people-centred mobilising approach had to be tackled carefully within the complex cultural context of Simbu. It necessitated conducting a culturally-adapted social market research (CASOMAR). Specific communities signalled their interest in entering into a dialogue with the project district teams, who sat down with them to find out what they saw as their own development priorities for agricultural development, marketing, income generation, vocational skills, communications problems, needs for health, literacy and women's development. As far as health needs were concerned, it emerged that in 40 mobilised communities, local people wanted knowledge and skills relating to hygiene in the household, improved food preparation and cooking practices, and knowledge and skills to prevent and treat common diseases. The project teams explained that community participation and contributions would be necessary as part of the activities which could be developed.

A.9 CULTURALLY-APPROPRIATE TRAINING IN RESPONSE TO COMMUNITY IDENTIFIED HEALTH NEEDS

A.9.1 A Novel Training Course

In March 1996, a six day multidisciplinary (health, literacy, agriculture, community development) training course for village health workers was held at a semipermanent/ bush material Lutheran community centre in one district. It was attended by 10 community-selected volunteers and six members of the government health staff who ran aid posts nearest to those villages. The district officers were actively involved. The multidisciplinary team had designed and prepared a range of participatory approaches as part of the flexible 'training package' developed for the course. Materials were to be mostly locally available at community level, or at least available in Kundiawa. The training team (two local training experts and the health adviser/facilitator) trained other trainers in literacy, community development, women's development to use a standard format for preparing the flexible 20 modules for teaching/learning sessions. The emphasis was on actively involving trainees and away from the often didactic teaching and learning methods customarily used. Teaching aids were prepared from locally available materials, such as a 'flannelgraph' (local blanket with cut-out, locally drawn coloured illustrations for nutrition teaching/ learning), demonstration model for births (locally made flexible cloth 'baby' and a cardboard box 'pelvis'), simple materials for a 'home delivery kit' and a couple of portable chalkboards.

A.9.2   Course Objective

The overall objective of the course was to set up a functional 'community-based microsystem' around the trained volunteer village health workers (VHWs) linked to local health staff at aid posts, and the district health centre. Corresponding objectives of the course were to train and equip volunteer VHWs to plan and lead specific health action in their own communities; stimulate action for personal and household hygiene, including attention to water and sanitation; know how to make the best use of local foods; use improved cooking methods and grow new vegetables; teach communities how to 'grow healthy children'; prevent community problems such as diarrhoea, and acute respiratory infections; promote immunisation; teach village women how to make and use homemade oral rehydration fluid; monitor child growth; promote and practice safe motherhood and improved new-born care; and, to be able to practice first aid skills.

A.9.3   Course Focus

The six-day course was designed to respond to the health-related needs discovered by means of CASOMAR among the 40 mobilised communities. Of the 74 needs identified, 43 per cent were health related, and 90 per cent fell within the social sector. The course was also designed around the needs of two types of participants, volunteer village health workers selected by their own village development committees, and local, two-year trained health staff from nearby aid posts. The objective of training two types of participants during a single course was to create the basis for a more sustainable and functional network, linking local communities and local health services. Although primarily trained for community-based work (unlike other types of health staff), the health staff had usually tended to remain in their health centres/aid posts, providing largely curative care. They were thus an under-utilised resource. By involving them in the training of the local VHWs they also had an opportunity for 'in-service' training themselves, although certain clinical and technical needs could not be matched during a course designed principally for VHWs.

A.9.4   Trainees Profiles

The VHWs were mostly female, most of them were married, from farming families, with 1–5 children, and most had attended primary school (one had attended secondary school). Several other interested observers from surrounding communities also attended the course unofficially. This indicated community interest. The aid post health staff were all married.

A.9.5   Course Content

During the first evening of the course (before the VHWs arrived), the training team held an informal session with local health staff in order to learn more about their working and living conditions, experience, interests and needs.

A.9.5.1   Getting to Know the VHWs

When training began, an early session involved a prepared list of questions used to stimulate answers and discussion with VHWs by using visual symbols on a matrix on the chalkboard. This exercise was also designed to focus the minds of participants on elements they would learn about during the course.

A.9.5.2   What Does a Family Need?

The next introductory exercise was 'What Does a Family Need?' This was a visual participatory exercise where a facilitator encouraged participants to draw an average family in the centre of the chalkboard. Then participants suggested basic needs that such a family had such as food, water, shelter, money, land and then health-related needs such as immunisation, care for pregnant women, treatment of common diseases and first aid. The exercise aroused lively interest among participants and observers. The main objective again was to focus on households. Key messages included *helt bilong famili* (healthy family) and *helt bilong komunitu* (healthy community). From this exercise emerged a clearer idea for participants about the purpose of their training and key future action areas.

A.9.5.3   Clean Body — Clean Home

On the second day of the course the emphasis, as requested by mobilised communities, was on *'Klin Bodi-Klin Haus'* (see Chart A. 2). This consisted of groupwork using 23 short key questions to discuss personal hygiene practices like washing daily, brushing teeth daily, changing clothes, attention to minor cuts, sleeping eight hours daily, using a toilet, and washing hands after using the toilet and before eating. Household hygiene and health practices included smoke escape mechanisms, availability of windows, adequate roof, pest control (mosquitoes, rats, cockroaches, flies), one toilet for every household, lid on the toilet hole, cutting long grass around the house, drainage of waste water, and fencing of pigs, chickens, goats, which are likely to devastate vegetable gardens. (Use of mosquito nets was mentioned later during the malaria session).

Chart A.2
Klin Body – Klin Haus (*) (Clean Body – Clean Home)

1. Wash body every day	...	11. Got cockroaches	...
2. Brush teeth every day	...	12. Got rats	...
3. Wash clothes often	...	13. Got mosquitoes	...
4. Sleep 8 hours	...	14. Use mosquito net	...
5. Eat 3 times a day	...	15. Long grass near house	...
6. Wash hands before eating	...	16. Got latrine (pit)	...
7. Wash hands after toilet	...	17. Latrine got cover	...
8. House has smoke hole	...	18. Got chicken pen	...
9. House has window	...	19. Got pig pen	...
10. Roof keeps out rain	...		

(*) Extracted from Feuerstein, M.T. (1997). *Poverty and Health - Regaining a Richer Harvest*, Macmillan, London.

A.9.5.4   Clean Drinking Water

This session was facilitated by the district health officer. He outlined the water supply situation in the district, water-related diseases/conditions (like diarrhoeal diseases, typhoid, scabies) and encouraged VHWs and health staff to help their communities to understand the importance of safe water. He outlined why water sources must be protected. He explained how to make an inexpensive *botol wara* (water bottle) constructed from a used and clean 2-litre plastic bottle, which could be used after using a latrine. One was hanging outside the latrine during the course. The next session was 'Stools Around the Place Cause Sickness' connecting water with sanitation. A key message was that programmes for clean water and sanitation must be considered and implemented together. A handout provided technical specifications for constructing and maintaining a pit latrine. Participants were helped to focus on diseases associated with inadequate disposal of human excreta like roundworms and told about the importance of washing hands after using the toilet, before cooking and breastfeeding.

A.9.5.5   Improved Nutrition

The afternoon session 'How To Make Best Use of Local Foods' began with the use of the locally made flannelgraph through which participants played a nutrition game, grouping local foods according to whether they mainly provided energy, protected against diseases, or stimulated physical growth. This led to a discussion about the traditional ways of preparing local foods, including steaming in bamboo. Then a female district agricultural officer introduced the session on 'Growing New Vegetables', discussing what participants already grew and how new vegetables could be introduced. This was followed by a cooking demonstration held in the open air. There were new recipes for making local dishes. The training team demonstrated how to make *'fis kaiks'* (sweet potato fish cakes), and savoury fried rice. Male participants were particularly interested in both recipes and the tasty outcomes, and participated in preparing both items, bemoaning the fact that they had never before had the opportunity to learn to cook as men do not customarily cook in Simbu.

A.9.5.6   Child Health

The third day began with a session on 'Growing Healthy Children'. The facilitator introduced participants to the normal growth pattern of a child from a foetus to five years of age. Pictures and flip charts were used to assist learning. Then signs of stunted growth and malnutrition were illustrated. Participants were introduced to the 'middle upper arm circumference' (MUAC) strip, which is a thin strip of plasticised paper specially marked and coloured to illustrate whether a child between 1–4 years is growing adequately, or if a degree of undernutrition/malnutrition is present. It is placed around the mid upper arm of a child 1–4 years of age. The colours reveal the nutritional status of the child. Each participant was shown how to colour and use their own MUAC strip in their own communities. Then each prepared their 'Report *buk bilong wok*' (report of my work) in a locally prepared personal exercise book, using three colours for monitoring the growth of children between 1–4 years in their own communities.

A.9.5.7   Preventive and Curative Treatment

The next session introduced participants to preventable diseases of childhood and the importance of immunisation for eligible children in their own communities. Pictures of diseases like measles, tetanus, polio, were distributed and discussed. The facilitator introduced a specially prepared immunisation matrix through which VHWs in liaison with community health workers (CHWs) and mother and child health (MCH) patrols can monitor the immunisation status of eligible children in their own communities. The last session of the morning introduced participants to common health problems in children, such as diarrhoea, fever and acute respiratory infections, and both preventive and simple curative action. An open-air practical session was held on the preparation of '*suga wara*' (sugar and boiled water) as rehydration therapy. Use of other liquids such as '*kau kau*' (sweet potato) water, rice water, guava leaf or papaya flower tea was also encouraged.

A.9.5.8   Safe Motherhood

The three afternoon sessions on safe motherhood and new-born care began with the session on *lukoutim gut bel mama* (safe and healthy pregnancy). During a participatory session the facilitator illustrated why ante-natal care is important, and what were some of the 'danger signs' (risk factors) which could be recognised at the community level during pregnancy. This led to discussion and demonstration of what preparations should be made in a household prior to home delivery. Within the official local government framework of encouraging facility-based deliveries, there is still a need, especially for women in remoter areas, to prepare better for deliveries which are likely to be at home. Participants discussed the contents of a simple home birth kit which costs 10 kina (around US $8) and consists of 9 items. It was pointed out that while a family will spend 40 kina to purchase items for the new-born, a similar amount spent on the mother is still not considered worthwhile. The simple home birth kit included cord ties, a new razor blade, soap, nail sticks, clean cloth for wiping the infant's eyes and mouth, a sanitary pad for the mother and a clean cloth to wrap the baby. Other items to be collected before the birth included a bucket, a water container, a hurricane lamp, firewood and a new *bilum* (locally woven traditional loose-weave bag) in which to wrap the baby. The newly introduced *Helt Buk Bilong Ol Meri* (women's health book) was also shown and the VHWs encouraged to ensure that women in their own communities obtained copies from the health services.

A.9.5.9   Birth and Postpartum Haemorrhage

The next session was preceded by an unusual role play. Two male participants enacted the role of a pregnant woman in labour and childbirth. Participants were obviously impressed by the implication that men could and should know far more than they did about childbirth. Then followed the session '*Helpim Mama Long Karim Gut Pikinini*' (clean and safe childbirth). The objective of the session was to learn what happens during a normal delivery, what can go wrong for the mother and the new-born, and what action to take. Facilitators conducted a lively session using the doll and box (originally prepared for the Safe Motherhood workshop in Kundiawa in 1995). They demonstrated the three stages of labour and delivery and immediate post-delivery requirements of the mother and the new-born. Post-partum haemorrhage was demonstrated using three bottles of red-coloured water to illustrate what was meant by heavy bleeding (the third bottle containing an amount which indicated heavy bleeding).

A.9.5.10   After Birth Care

The third session '*Lukoutim Gut Mama Behain Long Karim*' (good care after birth), aimed to teach VHWs and aid post health staff what the mother and the new-born needed after birth, how to recognise post-delivery 'danger signs' and what action to take. Again the doll and box were used as well as items from the simple home delivery kit. Participants were also shown a more extensive delivery kit consisting of 19 items which is planned for the trained village birth attendants (VBAs). Discussions followed on the benefits of breastfeeding, and appropriate ways to deal with cases where post natal danger signs appeared. Pictures were used to illustrate points made, but a flannelgraph would have been better. On the fourth day of the VHW training, there was a session on family planning, particularly for men, and on infertility problems.

A.9.5.11   Relevant Maps, Problems and Possible Solutions

At the beginning of the course, VHWs and aid post health staff had made a map (on locally purchased plastic sheeting) of the district, and marked out villages, aid posts, roads, location of the district office, health centre and literacy schools. Later, community development, agriculture and women's development activities were to be included on the map. The VHWs also made a basic health map of their own homeplace/workplace. Wider 'community mapping' may be introduced later. They also learnt how to refer patients to aid posts/health centre. They learnt basic first aid. On the final evening there was an in-depth discussion with the aid post health staff to summarise their needs which would enable them to function effectively in the VHW-Aid Post/ Health Centre 'microsystem'. At the moment they face multiple working and living problems. For example, at one aid post the only medical instrument available is a pair of scissors. At another, after sterilising instruments in a saucepan, the aid post staff has to wash the same saucepan and use it to cook the evening meal of sweet potatoes. Under such conditions it is not realistic to expect an adequate standard of care to be provided for safe motherhood or new-born care. Without basic equipment the health staff cannot even properly complete the mother's health record book, an important recent innovation for women's health in the province. There are plans of expansion, whereby such health staff will be enabled to purchase 12 essential medical instruments/items of equipment (real value 200 kina or US $312 for a subsidised price of 100 kina or US $156). Staff also need updated standard treatment manuals, and infant weighing scales. As aid post staff only earn 260 kina a month, and have families to feed, they have expressed willingness to pay 20 kina a month over 5 months. The instruments will be made available in a strong leather-look carrying case (actually a locally available bible case). Funds for the subsidy are being sought through Friends of PNG.

A.9.6   Course Evaluation

The VHWs and aid post staff were asked if they felt confident enough to apply what they had learnt in their own communities. All but three felt confident. Of those who did not, one had missed the first day of the course, one felt poorly integrated into his own community, and one health staff felt the need to have assistance in manning the aid post if he was to engage extensively in community work. Eighteen rated the course as the right length, and one as too short. Two participants said a visit to the local aid post should be included in the next course. The closing ceremony was attended by various dignitaries including the provincial assistant administrator who said that the course had 'gone directly to the heart of community problems'. Only with the participation of men and women at the community level can development really take place. He mentioned the planned 'rest house' system (an adaptation of previous colonial system where mobile extension teams visited local rest houses on a regular basis) to bring services closer to people. He said that the training course and development of a networking 'microsystem' was in line with this approach. It also could develop health leadership at the community level, with VHWs and local health staff playing a key role. He suggested a seventh training objective—to show caring and love for families and their well-being. Without love there can be no respect.

   The district manager said that the training course was the first of its kind held directly at the community level in the province. Overall the training course was considered to have achieved its objectives. A *mumu* (community feast) followed the closing ceremony. Since March 1987, VHWs have been trained in the five districts. This training has now been further adapted to be culturally-appropriate to local needs. The social marketing of health and development continues in Simbu despite many problems and challenges.

A.10   SOME OTHER EXAMPLES OF CULTURALLY-APPROPRIATE SOCIAL MARKETING IN SAFE MOTHERHOOD AND FAMILY PLANNING FROM ELSEWHERE

In relation to maternal health projects, social marketing has been described as the application of marketing principles to social programme design and management. It is a systematic attempt to introduce socially desirable objectives. In the context of health it relates to the adoption of health-promoting behaviour such as enhanced utilisation of services, trial and continued use of a product, and improvement of household or community practices. Social marketing provides a voice for the consumer—the programme beneficiaries— and is concerned with their perspectives and practices, making it easier for them to follow better practices.

A.10.1   Hospital Deliveries and the Mother's Privacy

For example, formative research revealed disparities between what the medical community and what pregnant women considered to be the quality of care at the clinic and hospital level in Cochabamba, Bolivia. Hospital deliveries were usually attended by several different medical professionals, including interns. But, pregnant women were adamant about having their privacy. Five phases of health communication activities were designed for policy-makers:

- Pregnant women and their health care providers.
- Advocacy for maternal health care and the quality of that care according to the perspective of the pregnant woman.
- Prenatal care.
- Clean and safe delivery.
- Post-partum and post natal care; and family planning.

Medical supervisors were oriented to the perspectives of pregnant women, and ways in which services and their staff could better meet their client's needs. Health care workers were given counselling training in each of these phases as part of this effort. Television and radio, clinic-based flip charts and community-based participatory activities were used and a '*vox populi*' (voice of the people) style in TV and radio spots was used to ask questions about danger signs. This resulted in women being better able to ask questions of their care providers.

Behaviour cannot be changed unless it is first understood. This is the basic rationale for conducting CASOMAR. Such research is conducted as part of programme design, using not only surveys and clinical data but also qualitative research that probes into the rationale for people's behaviour.

A.10.2   Different CASM Techniques

Many types of posters have been produced for promoting safe motherhood; some international for national and local adaptation, and some produced directly from local materials and by local designers. Pictures and photographs have also been used. To socially market safe motherhood among health care providers, a variety of technical guidelines and training modules exist, most prepared by WHO, as well as locally adapted checklists, such as the PNG example appended. Other culturally-appropriate training approaches and materials have included question and answer handouts for self-assessment, slides (such as the safe motherhood set available from TALC), and demonstrations, for example, of good practice. Culturally-appropriate social marketing of safe motherhood at the community level, bearing in mind the needs of non or minimally literate audiences, has included role plays, puppets, songs, and games. Videos have also been produced internationally and nationally.

In Nigeria a music video, by two well-known singers, asked Nigerians to choose the best time to have their children. In Mexico, audiences laughed at pregnant men in a hit television soap opera. In Turkey, a TV spot shows a popular comedian portraying a farmer dividing the family farm among his seven children: each gets only a pot of dirt. In Zimbabwe, a feature film tells the story of Rita, whose life as a student falls apart when she becomes pregnant.

A.11   CONCLUSION

In the case of the Papua New Guinea project, culturally-appropriate social marketing approaches included contacting communities to elicit their interest and commitment to joint action for development whose agenda was largely set by themselves. Culturally-appropriate approaches to safe motherhood included a two-pronged approach of listening to potential consumers in both communities and health services, in order to design responses matching their realities, needs and preferences. Unfortunately, a continuing climate of unrest and uncertainty continues to plague the province and the project. For example, health officers from provincial level have been deployed to districts without good provision for their living or working conditions. The provincial hospital is once again under central government control. Corrupt practices continue. The national health minister was sacked for reportedly misappropriating the equivalent of US $75,000, provincial politicians largely favour their own clans at the expense of others, and funds 'go missing' from a district revolving fund for community purchase of mosquito nets. Without sanctions and disciplinary action such practices may well continue. The project managers change, the constant presence of external review teams retards progress and complicates agreed upon project designs and objectives thus constantly 'moving the goalposts', and one funding agency suddenly withdraws financial support from the social section of the project, which includes the health component without warning. Fortunately, another donor may take it over, thus safeguarding the small but significant shoots which have began to sprout on the challenging cultural context of Simbu. Social unrest and tribal fighting continues, but by March 1996 a noticeable difference occurred, particularly in the town, when the government banned alcohol.

Cultural fragmentation necessitates adjustments of the project approach in each village/clan/valley/area. Basing training and action on identified community needs has increased community mobilisation, education and possibly sustainability. It took time to mobilise the 40 communities. But, evident community interest and mobilisation, indicate the cultural appropriateness of the approach taken.

A.12   RECOMMENDED READING

Gillett, J.E. (1990). *The Health of Women in Papua New Guinea*, PNG Institute of Medical Research.

International Labour Office (1995). *World Labour Report 1995*, ILO, Geneva.

National Sex and Reproduction Research Team and Carol Jenkins (1994). *National Study and Reproductive Knowledge and Behaviour in Papua New Guinea*, PNG Institute of Medical Research, Goroka, PNG.

Population Reports (1995). *Helping the News Media Cover Family Planning*, Series J, number 42, November.

——— (1989). *Light! Cameras! Action! Promoting Family Planning with TV, Video and Film*, Series J, number 38, December.

——— (1986). *Radio Spreading the Word on Family Planning*, Series J, number 32, September–October.

The Economist Intelligence Unit (1996). Pacific Islands: Papua New Guinea, Fiji, Solomon Islands, Western Samoa, Vanuatu and Tonga, *Country Report*.

Case Study B

The Bilekahalli Family Planning Project

Ajit Mani and Susan Thomas

B.1 INTRODUCTION

Although all names used in this case-study, including those of the project and it's staff are imaginary, it is based on a real-life family planning project in India, and illustrates some of the issues the project confronted during the 1980s and how it dealt with them.

B.1.1 The Population Problem in India

According to the 1991 census, the population of India was 844 million. There were 929 females per 1,000 males, and the female literacy rate was only 39.42 per cent against the rate of 63.86 per cent for males. Between 1921 and 1951, as high mortality was brought under control, there was a gradual rise in population. Between 1981 and 1991, India's annual compound population growth rate was 2.13 per cent. At this rate, the population is estimated to reach a billion by the year 2000. Just five of India's states—Uttar Pradesh, Bihar, Maharashtra, West Bengal and Andhra Pradesh—alone accounted for more than half the country's population.

There are strongly embedded attitudes in India towards marriage and procreation. Marriage and the raising of a large family are seen almost as religious responsibilities which will be rewarded by God.

The prejudice favouring male children is rooted in the belief that unless a man has a son to perform his last rites, he cannot attain *moksha* (salvation) in the other world. This prejudice is responsible for attitudes against female infants, girl children and women in general, to be found in most parts of India. Although there is a tendency now among urban communities to delay the marriage of girls till they are in their late twenties, eight out of 10 girls in India are married in their most fertile period—between 15 to 20 years of age.

There are a host of economic, social and cultural factors which encourage marriage at a relatively young age. Combined with the tradition of dowry and harassment by in-laws, many young women lead lives of misery with no control over their own lives. The Fertility Survey, conducted by the office of the registrar general of India in 1972, shows differential fertility rates on the basis of religious grouping.

Attitudes towards widow remarriage, divorce and confinement in the house of the girl's parents are some of the reasons cited for the relatively higher fertility in the Muslim community. Muslim personal law which

Pre-puberty Marriage

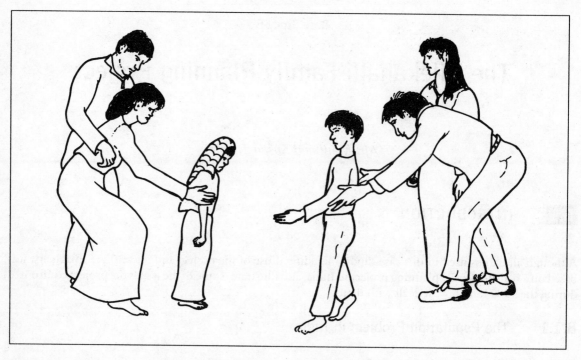

permits men to have more than one wife is yet another factor which distorts the otherwise common notion of a family unit consisting of a husband, a wife, and their children.

Although it is reported that in official circles there has been serious thinking about giving incentives to those who stop at one or two children and disincentives to those reproducing beyond this limit, there has been no political will in the country to translate this into legislation.

B.1.2   Government Response to the Problem

From the first Five-Year Plan, introduced in 1951, the Government of India launched the Family Planning Programme with the purpose of reducing the birth rate. India became the first country in the world to have a state sponsored population control programme for which a provision of Rs 6.5 million was made in the first Five-Year Plan.

The early clinical approach did not succeed in a largely illiterate society, and the programme was changed to a 'community extension' approach, which meant working with local structures and institutions. Contraceptive devices like the IUD (intra uterine device), introduced during the 1960s were not successful, and the government changed it's approach again to a 'camp approach', which emphasised sterilisation's and tubectomies.

During the Emergency period in India (1975–77), the country's Family Planning Programme suffered a serious setback when overzealous officials tried to speed up the programme. Many cases of brutality and excesses were reported, and it was not till the mid-1980s that the programme could be revived again, as the 'Family Welfare Programme'.

B.2 THE BILEKAHALLI RURAL PROJECT

The Bilekahalli Rural Project (BHRP) was one of the early voluntary efforts in India to tackle the population problem, by the Indian Institute of Family Planning (IIFP), India's premier family planning organisation.

The project was set up in the state of Karnataka, in south India, in a village a few kilometres outside the city of Bangalore. The population of Bilekahalli at the time (1986) was 64,000. The project manager was Mr Jay Krishna, and he had a team of 14 including an auxiliary nurse midwife.

The team moved into place quickly and divided the area into 12 sub-centres, consisting of 25 villages, each with an average population of 500. These 12 sub-centres were covered by 6 community welfare workers (CWWs).

B.2.1　A Baseline Survey

Conducting a baseline survey was the project manager's first task. He achieved this with the help of local school teachers and the unemployed youth in the village, so that the information would go back to the village. The baseline survey aimed to provide information about:

- Total population.
- Eligible couples (wife in the child-bearing age of 14–45).
- Total acceptors of family planning methods.
- Village profile.
- Institutions in the village.
- Youth clubs, women's groups (*mahila mandals*).
- Medical facilities.
- Water resources.
- Education levels of couples.
- Literacy levels in the village.

The survey divided couples into:

(*a*) **Primary sterility couples**—couples married for more than five years who have not had any children.

(*b*) **Priority couples**—newly married couples who do not have children yet, and couples who have three or more children.

(*c*) **Two-child couples**—couples who have two children already or are expecting their second child.

B.2.1.1　Results of the 1986 Baseline Survey

The results were quite striking:

Literacy levels in the area were very low—i.e., 25 per cent overall and only 12 per cent of women were literate.

Family planning acceptors constituted only 15–20 per cent of the married women. These female acceptors were mostly in the group which had more than three children. In such cases, tubectomy was the preferred method.

Infant mortality in the area was 78 per 1000 live births.

Average age at marriage was 18–19 years for boys and 14–15 years for girls.

Average family size was 10 members for joint families and 7–8 members for nuclear families.

Family size analysis showed that:

10 per cent were single child families.

40 per cent were two-children families.

50 per cent were families with three or more children.

B.2.2   Problems Faced in the Early Phase of the Project

The first inquiries clearly indicated the strong impact of cultural factors on villagers' fertility behaviour.

At first, people closed their doors when the IIFP jeep came to the village. The old people were outraged. How could these senseless city people come to the village to talk about something as personal and almost religious as having children? How could anyone talk about sex? Only the drunken truck drivers on the highway near Bilekahalli and the painted prostitutes, with strands of jasmine flowers in their hair, talked about sex and laughed aloud without any shame.

One of the ladies in the IIFP team wore a low cut blouse revealing much of her body. Another member of the team was a young girl, just out of college. What did she know about child bearing, or dealing with husbands who worked hard in the fields?

Only about 10 years ago, during the Emergency, many men had vasectomies performed on them, and they remembered the case of Raja Gowda who had died during the operation. It was rumoured that if men were 'operated' upon, they would no longer be men and would not be able to perform the duties of a husband. Men would become weak and tired while they were still young, and children would throw stones at them when they walked along the dusty streets.

Children were necessary to look after parents in their old age, and a son was absolutely essential to light the funeral pyre of his father. How else could a man go to heaven?

The men were not interested in talking to the volunteers and staff from the IIFP. They were too busy in the fields. It was the women who first agreed to undergo the tubectomy operations. Mr Jay Krishna, the manager, found after 6 months that the majority of women who volunteered for the operation were those who already had 3 or more children. They came forward for the operation so that their husbands would not have to be operated upon. According to religious tradition, the devoted wife (*pativrata*) could snatch her husband from the demons of hell and take him up to heaven, just as the snake catcher drags the snake from it's hole by force.

B.3   THE PROJECT STRATEGY

The socio-cultural data that emerged from the initial investigation provided the basis of the subsequent project strategies.

B.3.1   Target Segmentation

Jay Krishna knew that the first thing he had to do was to segment the target population by dividing the village population into socially recognisable and meaningful groups. This would enable the project to develop specific programmes for each group. Accordingly, boys were organised into *yuvak mandals* (youth clubs) and girls into *yuvathi mandals* (young women's clubs). Women in the child-bearing age group were organised into *mathru sanghas* (mothers' clubs).

Target Segmentation

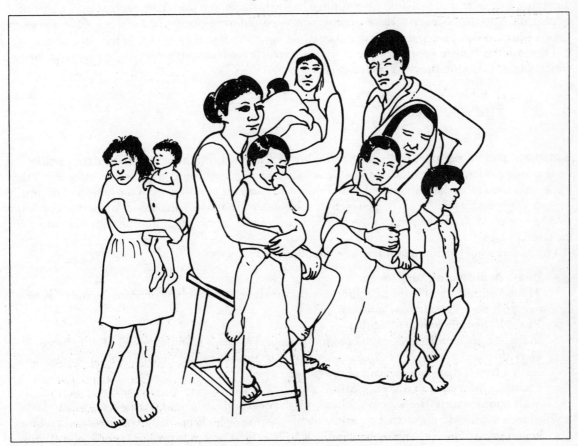

B.3.2   Identification of Local Resources

The project manager knew that he could not achieve his goals with the help of a team of staff from Bangalore. He looked around to see what local resources he could find in order to multiply the reach of the Bangalore team. At the same time, he transferred his rather young female assistant to the office and employed an older lady in her place. He also issued instructions about appropriate clothing and behaviour for field staff.

The *dais* (traditional birth attendants) were identified as key influencers in the project strategy. They were oriented to the programme and they agreed to talk to groups of villagers on the subject of sexuality and reproductive biology. The *dais* were given a special kit to use when they attended deliveries. They were taught to use brand new razor blades to cut the umbilical cord instead of their pocket knives which they also used for cutting betel nuts.

The educated unemployed youth were also co-opted into the programme. They were frustrated that although they had broken with tradition and completed their school education and had even attended university, they were unable to find jobs. Although they had acquired university degrees, they were unable to compete with the boys and girls of the city, who appeared to be getting all the jobs. What was worse, having educated themselves, they felt that they could not go back to the hard life of the field.

These educated unemployed saw the project as a vehicle for finding meaningful employment through which they could regain their lost pride.

B.3.3   Strategic Planning

With the help of his expanded team, Jay Krishna began planning his strategies. In those days, participatory rural appraisal (PRA) was unknown as a methodology, and the team instead visited each village over a three week period, to talk to the villagers and communicate to them the overall goals of the project. This usually evoked a lively discussion, which helped identify the quarters from which maximum support or opposition could be expected. It also helped to suggest appropriate methods of communicating with and influencing the target groups.

The project would go through three different phases as follows:

- **Phase A: Softening-up process**
  The team decided that in the first three months they would use a variety of processes and platforms to expose the villagers to key information.
- **Phase B: Social change attempts**
  In the next six months, programmes to influence and re-shape attitudes would be introduced.
  Only after this, a number of programmes would be introduced to consolidate the campaign and create a lasting change in the lives of the villagers.
- **Phase C: Information dissemination**
  Mass contact activities were organised with the help of the educated unemployed youth. Local women politicians, the district superintendent of police (who happened to be a woman) and the headmistress of the girls high school in Bilekahalli were requested to preside over these functions. This eased the tension considerably, and the village women found that sex and reproduction were not such taboo subjects, after all.
  Film shows on the biological aspects of reproduction were organised, and provided a good diversion in the evening.
  Family planning posters began to appear at the places where villagers gathered in the evenings, and boxes of NIRODH brand condoms began to be displayed prominently in all the petty shops and provision shops in the villages.

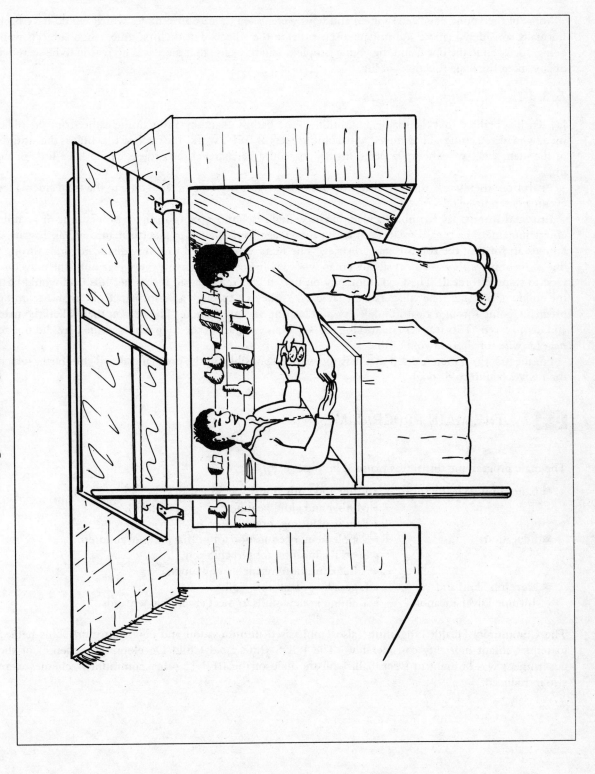

Some of the young educated women and boys were asked to introduce topics which would have been normally considered taboo, and initiate discussions in the village. For the first time, taboo subjects were being discussed in the open, and the young people began to realise that there was no reason to be secretive or shy about the basic functions of life.

B.3.3.1   Changing Attitudes

Jay Krishna realised that the major opposition to the Family Planning Programme came from the older men, who were getting a bit annoyed with some aspects of IIFP's work. He realised that unless the attitude of the men, who were the main decision-makers, could be changed the project would have little or no impact.

Apart from their work, the men had little or no interest in anything except going to the local cinema for evening entertainment.

Entertainment: Jay Krishna decided that he would reach these men through a programme of evening entertainment. As a special treat, the men in the village were invited to a performance of Yakshagana, a famous art form of the south Kanara district. The men were exposed to a very disturbing idea through one of these plays. It was a story about a man whose wife became pregnant every year until she prayed to God to stop her ordeal. The Gods took pity on her and decreed that in future her husband would bear the children, not she. The villagers were shocked as they sat through a performance of a man becoming pregnant, going through a painful delivery, and bearing an ugly demon. The demon then killed the man and disappeared. This was very disturbing indeed. Ramesh, one of the men who saw the play, did not go near his wife for almost two months!

For the first time, men realised that they too were responsible for the pregnancies and childbirths which their wives had to go through.

B.4   THE MAIN PROGRAMME

The main programme thrust was planned in three sectors:

- ■ Community Health:
  - • Water and sanitation.
  - • Mother and child health.
  - • Family planning services.
- ■ Education:
  - • Supplementary education for primary school children.
  - • Special education for girl children.
  - • Adult education for men and women.
- ■ New Job Skills and Income Diversification:
  - • Upgrading of existing skills.
  - • Training in new skills to meet emerging demands.

The Community Health Programme also emphasised immunisation and child nutrition. This helped to reduce infant mortality considerably. The ICDS (Integrated Child Development Scheme) of the government was brought to Bilekahalli with the help of the IIFP. 12 other community schemes were also introduced.

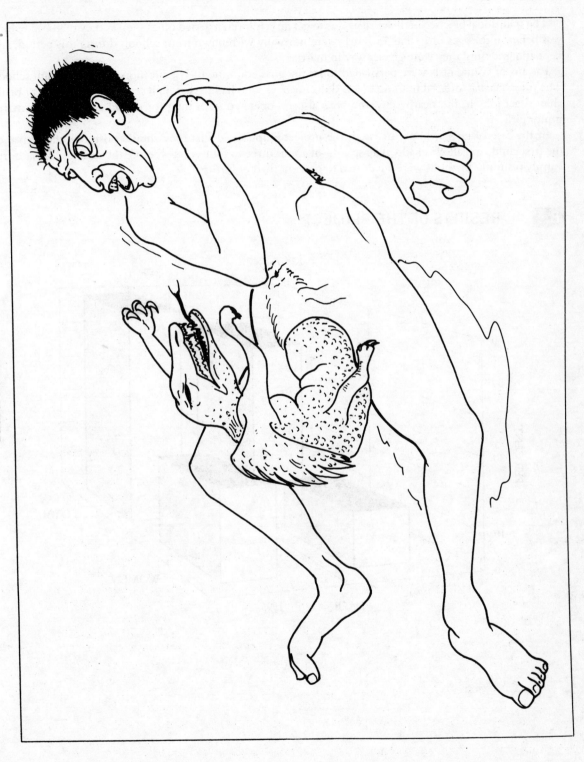

Birth of a Demon

The traditional practice in the villages was to get girl children married off as soon as they matured, which was between the ages of 13 and 15. Girls were normally withdrawn from schools during this period, and kept at home until they were given away in marriage.

Parents of young girls were persuaded to let the girls continue their education at least till high school. The *yuvak mandals* offered training in job skills for boys who had passed high school. In the hope of being able to get jobs in the nearby city, the boys also co-operated with the project and agreed not to marry minor girls.

In the case of girls who got married, the project emphasised that they should postpone the arrival of the first child, and allow an adequate space—of about three to four years—before the next child was born. Family planning methods were advocated to prevent further births.

B.5   RESULTS OF THE PROJECT

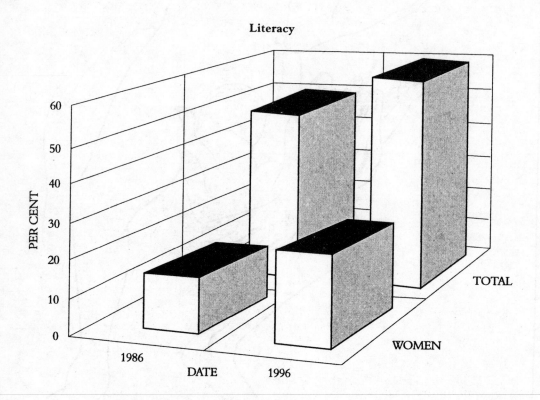

Acceptance of Family Planning Methods

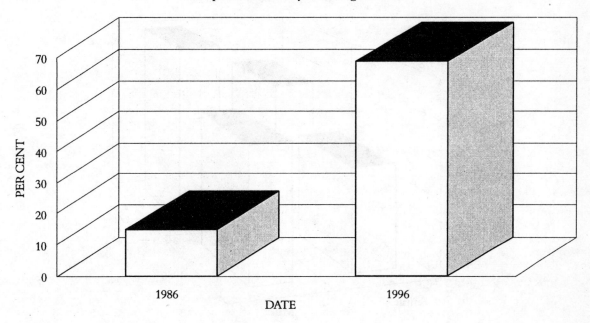

Infant Mortality

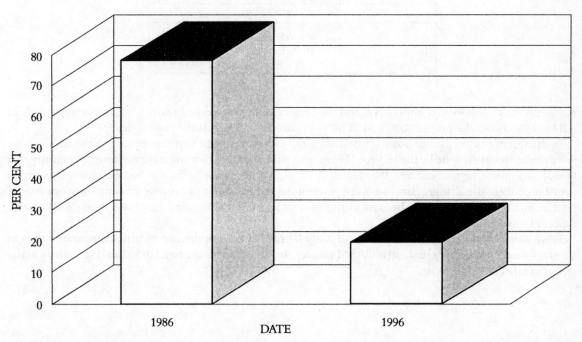

Age at Marriage

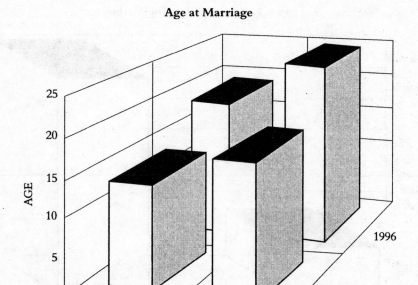

	Average family size	
	1986	1996
Joint	10 members	N.A.
Nuclear	7–8	5.5

Although the results looked impressive, and the project team had worked really hard, it was impossible to tell how successful the project had been. This is because of a defect in the project design.

In the absence of any comparison, it was difficult to justify the claim that the changes in the tables above were due to the work done by the project. There was, after all, a consciousness throughout the country that family size should be reduced and the slogan, 'A small family is a happy family' had become a byword all over India. Were the changes that had taken place in the villages due to a process of maturation or history? Jay Krishna would never know because at the time of starting his project he had not thought about this aspect of project measurement.

From a theoretical point of view, this case study highlights the importance of truly comparative data to substantiate the impact of a particular CASM project. It also indicates the need of cultural sensitivity at the outset of any CASM exercise.

Case Study C

A Two Year Mother-child Health Pilot Project at Loja, Ecuador, South America

Patricio Mora

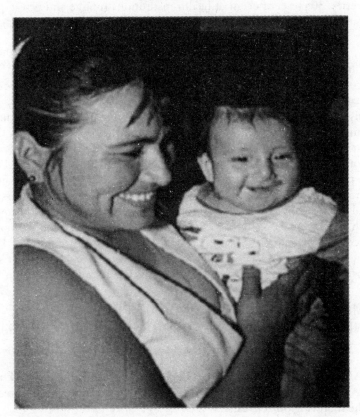

C.1   THE SOCIO-CULTURAL SETTING

In the mountains of southern Ecuador, women wait for their 'change of life' (menopause) as a kind of family planning. Families of 10 children are the average and no one escapes poverty. It is common for women and children to die unnecessary and preventable deaths.

C.1.1   The Population Problem in Loja, Ecuador

The fertility rate in Loja (4.15) is above the national average (3.61) and the use of family planning methods is lower than the national average (44.8 *versus* 56.8). In Loja, the methods most used are tube ligation (12.5 per cent), IUD (9.5 per cent), calendar (9.5 per cent), coitus interruptus (5.1 per cent). These methods are promoted mainly by the Ministry of Health (MOH), health centres, private medical practitioners and NGOs. There is a great, unsatisfied demand for family planning methods. 67.6 per cent of mothers, whose youngest child is under two years of age, did not want to have more children. They were not, however, using any contraceptive methods.

The maternal mortality rate in Loja is an estimated 210 per 100,000 live-births. The main causes of mortality are: haemorrhage, infection and pregnancy's hypertensive disease.

Of all birth deliveries, 30 per cent occur at health institutions (public and private). The remaining 70 per cent take place at home with the assistance of traditional birth attendants (TBAs), family members or with no help at all.

Ecuador is largely a Catholic country. In rural areas, religion is important in family planning decisions; most of the counselling of rural communities is done by the priest during confession. The Catholic Church dismisses modern contraceptives and favours natural methods. However, during focus group discussions it was discovered that couples were unsure about the proper use of natural methods.

An interesting discovery was the fact that during the harvesting of sugarcane in the coastal region, there is a seasonal migration of men, who seek to supplement their incomes, from the Highlands to the sugarcane fields. In Ecuador, prostitution is legal and sexually transmitted diseases (STDs) are a major health problem among men from the Highlands who migrate seasonally. In the late 1970s and early 1980s there was a massive public health campaign in Ecuador focusing on the use of condoms to prevent STDs. Therefore, men perceive the use of condoms as a means of preventing the transmission of STDs during extramarital sex, and dislike using condoms with their wives for moral reasons. Many men would tell us: 'I use condoms with prostitutes, how could I use it with my wife, she is clean!'. Another cultural barrier to the use of contraceptives is the male fear of their wives' infidelity. A man will say 'I'm away from home during the sugarcane season, if my wife uses contraceptives she is free to do whatever she wishes and I will never know it'. This pattern of thinking obviously posed a threat to our family planning programme.

 C.2   THE MOTHER-CHILD HEALTH PILOT PROJECT AT THE ESPINDOLA AND PALTAS CANTONS, PROVINCE OF LOJA

In March 1996, **PLAN INTERNATIONAL (ECUADOR)**, the **United Nations Fund for Population Activities (UNFPA)** and the **Ecuador Ministry of Health (MOH)**, signed an agreement for a two year Pilot Project with the following objectives:

- **To strengthen the technical and management skills of the Espindola and Paltas health areas by:**
  - Strengthening community participation in the diagnosis and effective solution of the population's reproductive problems.
  - Strengthening of joint planning and implementation of activities between communities and MOH.

- **To improve coverage and quality of health services by:**
  - Satisfying the families' reproductive preferences.
  - Lowering maternal deaths caused by haemorrhage, infections, miscarriage and pregnancy's hypertensive disease.
  - Increasing the early detection of breast and cervical cancer.

PLAN INTERNATIONAL, as the institution responsible for project implementation, hired the Pilot Project manager, who then recruited a team which includes: six community health facilitators, two supervisory nurses, one training co-ordinator, one information-communication co-ordinator and one accountant.

The project manager, training co-ordinator, information-communication co-ordinator and the accountant are located in Loja to co-ordinate actions with the provincial department of health. The supervisory nurses co-ordinate actions with the health area managers. The community health facilitators co-ordinate actions with the staff of 14 rural health centres as well as with 96 community health providers.

The team began work in April 1996 by promoting the project among the MOH staff at Loja as well as at the health areas of Espindola and Paltas. The team also asked permission of more than 300 community leaders for project implementation in their respective communities. Only general information was given so as to avoid 'contaminating' the sample for the survey yet to come.

The field team was trained and it then conducted a cluster baseline sample survey among mothers whose children were under two years of age. The information was collected with the assistance of community leaders, who asked mothers to remain at home during the research and MOH's staff who implemented and supervised the survey. It took about two months to complete the survey.

C.2.1   Main Results of the Baseline Survey

- **Prenatal care**
  - 56 per cent had received prenatal care from medically-trained personnel.(★)
  - 21 per cent had received prenatal care from an assistant nurse.
  - 35 per cent had received prenatal care from a TBA.
  - 23 per cent had received no prenatal care.

- **Birth delivery care**
  - 30 per cent was attended by medical personnel.(★)
  - 34 per cent was attended by a TBA.
  - 35 per cent was attended by a family member.
  - 1 per cent was not attended by anyone.

- **Family planning**
  - 89 per cent does not want any more children.
  - 32 per cent does not want any more children and use family planning methods.
  - 68 per cent does not want any more children and use NO FP method, i.e., there is an unmet demand for family planning methods.

- **Cancer in women (knowledge of the Papanicolaou test)**
  - 77 per cent did not know of the test for detection of cervical cancer.

- 8 per cent thought that the test was to test for infection.
- 15 per cent knew that the test was for the detection of cervical cancer.

(★) Even though most women go to the health centre for prenatal care, for cultural reasons they prefer to deliver at home. Women in rural areas deliver their babies by kneeling and grabbing a hanging rope; they are not accustomed to the Westernized way of delivery implemented in health centres, i.e., to deliver in a horizontal posture.

C.2.2 Culturally-adapted Feedback of the Survey Results to the Communities

Once the survey had been conducted, the team designed a simple way of giving the information back to the participating communities. A pamphlet was distributed with icons showing the findings as follows:

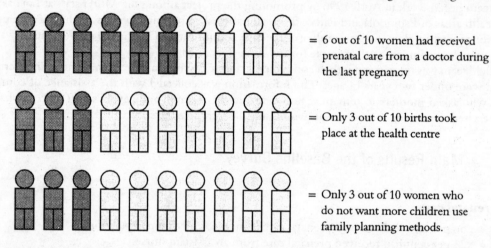

= 6 out of 10 women had received prenatal care from a doctor during the last pregnancy

= Only 3 out of 10 births took place at the health centre

= Only 3 out of 10 women who do not want more children use family planning methods.

These pamphlets were discussed at community assemblies. The participants were asked to show their understanding by presenting the findings in their own way. They used flowers (red flowers represented the population who took care of themselves and the less colourful represented the population at risk), they also used oranges, limes and coloured sticks to represent the people.

C.3 SELECTION AND RECRUITMENT OF COMMUNITY HEALTH PROVIDERS

The selection criteria of suitable communities were as follows:

- Communities with no health centre.
- Communities with no access to public transportation.

During the initial meetings for promoting the Pilot Project, the team asked the community leaders to select candidates who would be then interviewed by the project and MOH staff. The recommended profiles of suitable candidates were:

- Previous community volunteering history, preferably in health.
- The person must be a community resident for at least five years.
- The age should range between 25 and 45.
- They should be married.
- Preferably successful users of family planning methods.
- Traditional birth attendants.
- Community healers or traditional medicine practitioners.
- Community personnel trained previously by the MOH.
- People who had time available to undergo training.
- Preferably people who knew how to read and write Spanish.
- All candidates must appear with a document signed by community leaders showing that their candidacy has been agreed democratically in a community assembly.

Some of the potential candidates withdrew when they learnt that volunteers would not get any pay or special perks. 241 candidates were sent. All of them were interviewed by relevant project and MOH staff, who were from the closest rural health centre to the community from which the candidate was sent. 98 were recruited as community health providers (CHP) out of the 241 interviewed. All CHPs participated in the feedback of the baseline survey results.

C.4 COMMUNITY ACTION CYCLE

Once the people knew in terms of numbers what was happening within their social context, the Pilot Project staff began by training the MOH personnel and the CHPs about conducting a community action cycle. The community action cycle (CAC) involves a qualitative investigation into reproductive health. This cycle has four phases:

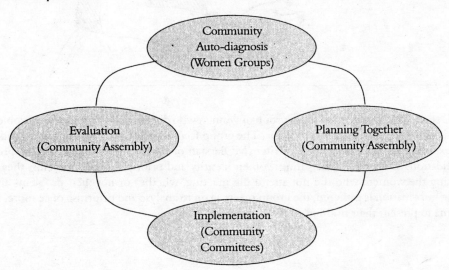

C.4.1 Auto-diagnosis

Self-diagnosis

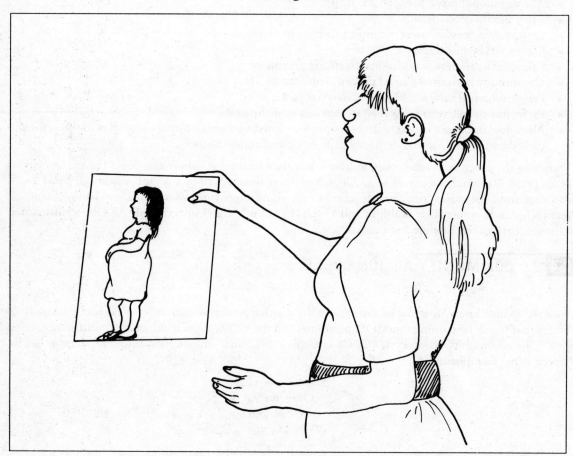

The CAC starts with an extended focus group of women who discuss their reproductive problems aided by drawings displaying reproductive problems. The group facilitator (a CHP) asks questions and leads the women to express their opinions, while a writer (MOH staff or a school teacher) records the proceedings for later validation. Once the participating women identify and prioritise their problems, they go door-to-door asking the women, who did not attend the meeting, whether or not their problems are similar. When all the information is gathered, the group meets again to analyse and prioritise once more. They use a socio-drama to present their findings to the community assembly.

C.4.2   Planning Together

Planning together

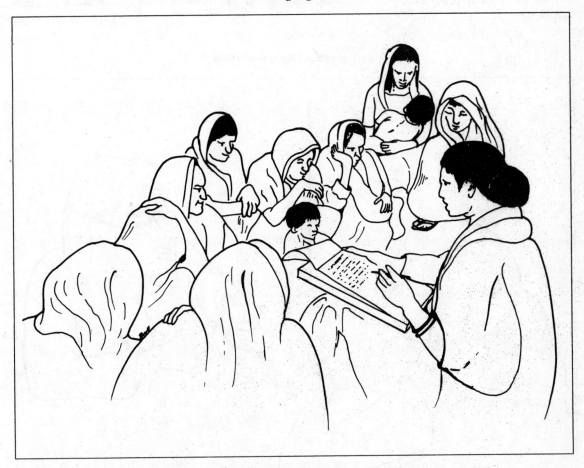

Community leaders, opinion leaders, priests, teachers and local authority representatives are all invited to this meeting. The assembly jointly identifies cultural barriers that interfere with the reproductive safety of families, all of which are recorded. The assembly then proceeds to prioritise their problems and develops a **plan of action** to solve the problems in a matrix as follows:

Reproductive problem	Identified barrier	Proposed action(s)	Who are to perform the activities	Starting date

At the end of the meeting a document which includes the community plan of action is read and signed by all participants (some communities even notarise such a document).

C.4.3   Implementation

The women's group holds a monthly follow-up meeting and reports to the assembly about the progress achieved.

Action cycle: Implementation

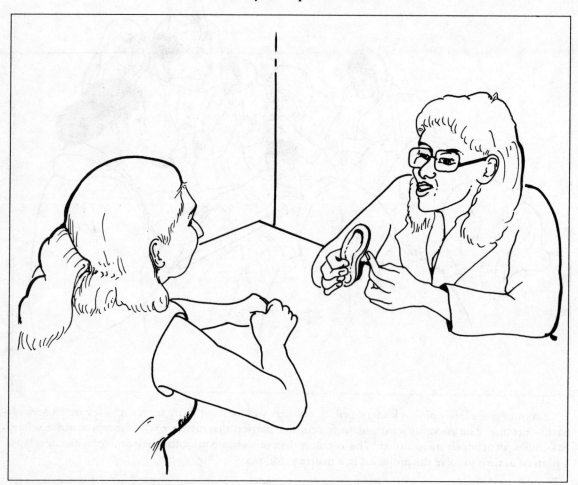

C.4.4   Evaluation

Each year, the community gets together to analyse the outcome of their plan of action and to develop a new community action cycle.

Action cycle: Evaluation

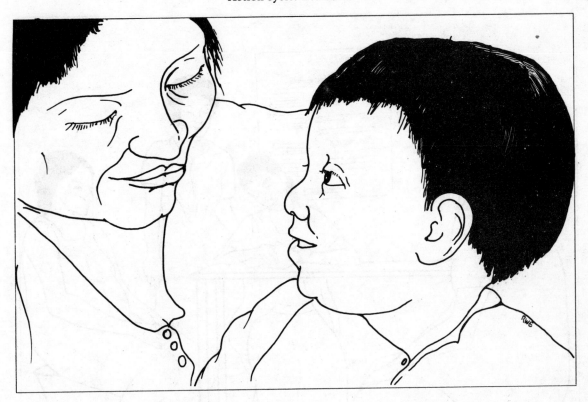

C.4.5   Findings of the CAC

Reproductive Problem	Identified Barriers	Proposed Action(s)	Who are to Perform these Activities	Starting Date
Mother with large family	• Fear of religion • Lack of knowledge about family planning options	• To talk with the priest • Family planning workshops	• Committee of leaders and teachers • MOH staff, CHP	• 1 January 1997 • 1 February 1997
Haemorrhage	• Domestic violence	• Workshop on human relations	Priest and/or teachers	15 January 1997
Infection	• No one takes care of mothers after birth	• Home visits after birth delivery	CHP, MOH staff	1 January 1997
Death due to reproductive emergencies	• Poverty	Fund-raising for credits for reproductive emergencies	Women's group	1 January 1997

At the Health Centre

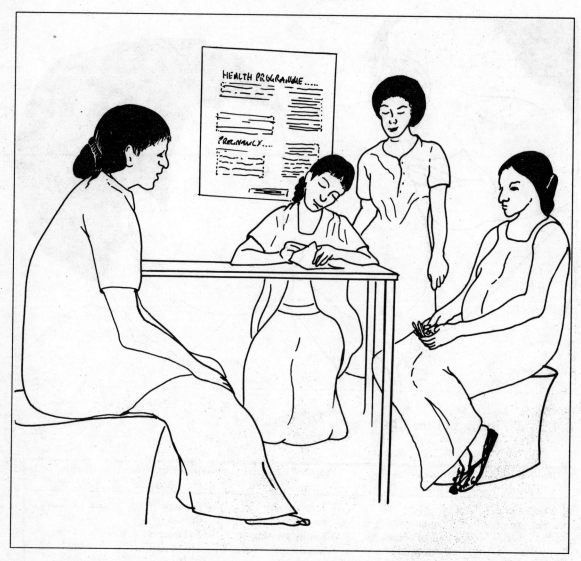

14 months after the start of the project there were already as many as 61 organised and functioning women's groups, which acted as encouragement for other women to follow the model of the women's group.

C.5   PROJECT STRATEGIES

The overall strategy of this project is part of a strategy for the South America region within PLAN INTERNATIONAL that focuses on three main areas:

- **Health promotion** which involves culturally-adapted social marketing. It provides information, education and communication on the project's interventions.
- **Improvement of quality of services** to meet consumers' demand created by the promotional activities, such as for instance the supply of knowledge and means of family planning, provision of adequate equipment, public health facilities and community health posts.
- **Professional training for MOH staff and continuous education for CHP**, the training curricula being approved by the local university and national government.

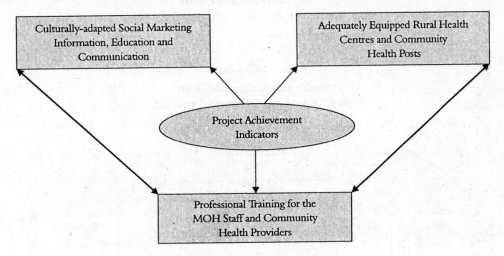

C.5.1   Establishment of a Community Health System

The project's main challenge was to establish a health management system based on community participation. Prior to the onset of the project, the MOH's organisational structure focused on the provider rather than on the consumer of health services.

Figure C.1
Conventional MOH Organisational Structure

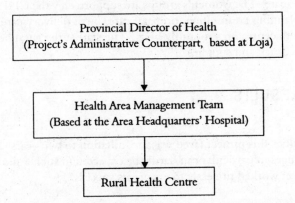

The project proposed a different approach: it includes community actors as an important part of a dynamic system of health service delivery. The revised structure has already been successfully implemented:

Figure C.2
Revised MOH Organisational Structure

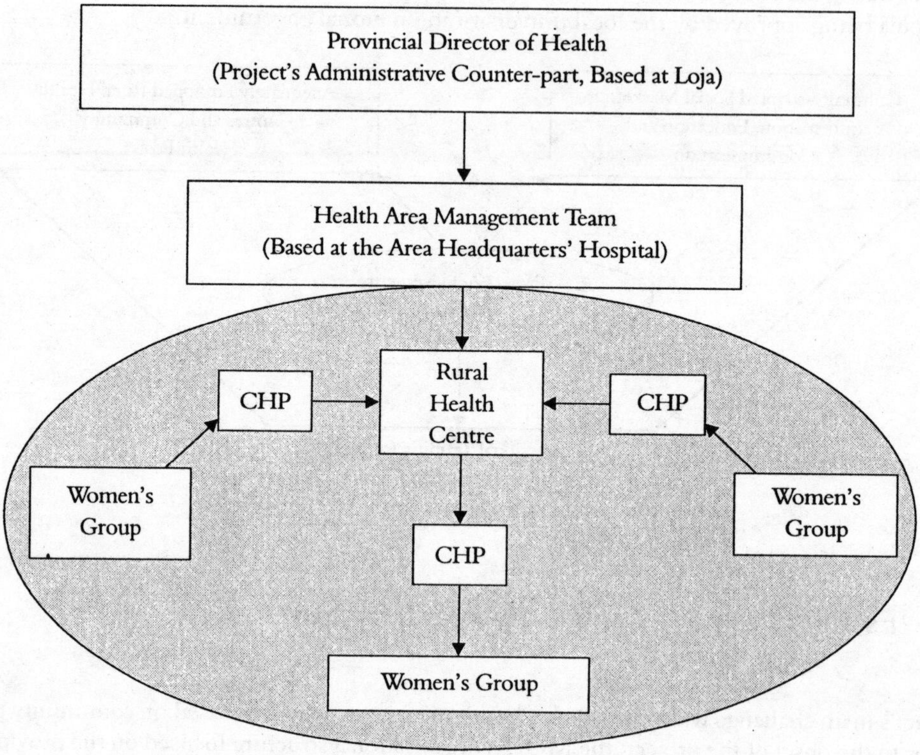

The shadowed area represents a **community health system**, in which community health providers (CHP) and women's groups participate. The women's groups are supported by the CHPs who report the outcome of their services (family planning counselling, prenatal care, birth delivery care, post-natal care and first aid services) to a rural health centre on a monthly basis. The staff at the rural health centre supervise and provide the CHPs with feedback and supplies.

C.6   PROJECT RESULTS

One of the greatest difficulties this project faced was its limitation to two years. Significant social changes in general and fertility changes in particular can hardly be expected in such a short period, even though all those involved in the project worked tirelessly to ensure its success.

C.6.1   Achievements Up to Date

- Establishment of 16 community health systems.
- Selection and recruitment of 96 community health providers.
- Establishment of 96 community health posts.
- Organisation of 61 women's groups.
- Design of a manual for culturally-adapted standards of service delivery for the various structural levels (i.e., hospitals, rural health centres and community health posts). This manual has already been adopted by the MOH.
- A manual of protocols for supervising the quality of service delivery, taking into account the differences pertaining to the various structural levels.
- A computerised information system (Epiinfo and EXEL) for monitoring service delivery has been installed. This system was designed by the local university and has been adopted by the MOH.
- A computerised system for government accounting has been installed in the two health areas.
- A community network of 100 social communicators, for local production of radio programmes for health promotion, has been established.
- Two adolescent theatre groups, for health promotion have been set up.
- One promotional video—IN OUR OWN WORDS—has been produced.

C.6.2   Challenges

- The two year time-frame of the project is too short.
- The MOH is not ready yet to take over the project without assistance.
- The CHPs and mothers' groups have more rapport with the project than with the MOH staff, which makes the fading out of the project difficult.
- Religion is still a big obstacle in securing the impact of modern family planning methods.
- The computerised information system is still in the validation process.
- The computerised accounting system has to be up-dated with recent governmental policy changes.
- In the Paltas health area, the personnel work on short-term contracts only; there is thus a risk of losing trained staff.

C.7   CONCLUSION

The most valuable part of the project have been the nurses contracted by PLAN INTERNATIONAL; they trek long distances over difficult terrain to each community to increase health awareness. The assistance of the contracted staff is invaluable in co-ordinating the roles of locally elected CHPs, MOH doctors, nurses and their assistants and thereby ensuring project sustainability.

Culturally-adapted social marketing has proved a great asset in helping the project achieve what it did. By practising careful target segmentation, different approaches were used for the different parties involved in the project, such as women, priests and MOH staff. Pictures of members of the community have been used rather than drawings for educational materials; cards and bingo games with messages relating to reproductive health are used by women's groups for income generation during community meetings and festivities.

In spite of the myth that government institutions are reluctant to change, co-ordinating the project with the MOH has been a rewarding experience. NGOs working in the health area are well-advised to realise that their role is to provide the MOH with attractive options and leave it to the government to decide whether and which of the changes to adopt.

Case Study D

A Community Self-help Programme in Kenya and Other Examples of the Use of CASM Relating to HIV/AIDS/STD

Marie-Therese Feuerstein and Anne Owiti

D.1 INTRODUCTION

In the field of health, there are two specific areas where culturally-appropriate social marketing has been particularly useful. The first is family planning, where various developers have approached their target audience in the same way as businesses approach their potential customers, and the second is the area of HIV/AIDS/STD (Human immuno-deficiency virus/acquired immuno-deficiency syndrome/sexually transmitted diseases), which has, from the start, extensively pursued a wide range of social marketing approaches and techniques. This case study is presented in two parts.

The first part outlines how and why an AIDS/HIV self-help programme has been rapidly developing in a Nairobi slum area. The programme is spearheaded by Anne Owiti, a Kenyan nurse who has facilitated the emergence of a dynamic, culturally-appropriate, home-based care programme within a challenging context of constant change. The second part outlines experiences from other parts of the world where culturally-appropriate social marketing techniques have been developed in response to the challenges faced by HIV/AIDS/STDs.

D.2 THE SOCIO-CULTURAL CONTEXT OF THE PROGRAMME

Kibera is the largest slum area in Nairobi, Kenya. It is home to a multi-cultural population of around 700,000 people living in 13 villages. The emergence of HIV/AIDS worsened the already poor health situation and problems in the area. It is estimated that around 25 per cent of the population is HIV positive. Kibera lacks proper infrastructure, hence the lack of adequate clean water and proper sanitary disposal of human excreta. There are about six water mains running through Kibera, and most people purchase their water from the water kiosks which are owned by individuals. Water and sanitation related diseases are very common. Parents seek medical help only in the most serious of cases.

Most people seek work: 99 per cent of the population is unemployed; only one per cent are employed as barmaids in the informal sector, consisting mainly of unregistered shops and factories. Many are self-employed (trading, selling services, working as casual labourers in simple construction or manufacturing ventures). Because of lack of vocational training and low literacy and numeracy, it is hard for them to move into the formal sector where incomes are higher and job security is enhanced. Therefore incomes tend to remain low and insecure.

It is not known how many people live below the poverty line. Non-government agencies, who work in the area, have drawn attention to the fact that growing poverty is increasing the number of multiple-partner situations involving various forms of sexual patron-client relationships. The fragmentary data suggests that relationships with prostitutes play a significant role in the spread of sexually transmitted diseases (STDs) and HIV/AIDS in both urban and rural areas, and between a third to over half of the prostitutes may be infected with an STD at any time. Transmission of HIV continues as other prostitutes and wives are infected. The low cultural and socio-economic status of women facilitates the heterosexual spread of STDs and HIV infection in urban areas. At the same time, the spread of HIV/AIDS threatens to erase whatever progress that has been made in raising the status of women, by tying them to their caring roles. This further limits their access to education and income-generating activities.

D.3 ORIGIN OF THE KIBERA SELF-HELP PROGRAMME (KSHP)

In September 1993, a Kenyan nurse-midwife, with the help of ACTIONAID, started the Kibera Self-help Programme. Kenya was late in accepting that HIV/AIDS was a problem, unlike countries like Uganda and Zambia. The increasing number of AIDS orphans was the main stimulus for the programme. Another, was the realisation that slum dwellers had little or no access to home-based care, counselling and support. The nurse-midwife had encountered people in need of such services and support at her newly established private practice. She then turned her attention to the overwhelming need of slum dwellers for appropriate and accessible care. Underpinning the programme is a commitment to the creation of a society that is fair and just, in which all people lead a harmonious life.

D.4 PROGRAMME PHASES

D.4.1 Culturally-adapted Social Market Research (CASOMAR)

As a preliminary to raising public awareness of the existence and dangers of the spread of HIV/AIDS, it was necessary to begin with a stock-taking exercise of attitudes, values and beliefs surrounding sexuality. A few key cultural variables such as lifestyle, sexuality norms, secrecy surrounding HIV/AIDS and confidentiality were first identified and then explored to form the basis of compiling a cultural profile of the target community. This profile indicated that unemployment and widespread poverty lead to a high divorce rate because men cannot support their families; they also lead to a lot of casual sex. Most young people have nothing to do. This makes them engage in sexual activities early in life. CASOMAR revealed that most 15 year old boys and girls already had sex more than a 100 times. These young people explained that they prefer to die of AIDS in five to ten years rather than die of hunger, which they see as the only alternative. Prostitutes pointed out that they too face the same dilemma: to die young either of AIDS or of starvation. Various CASOMAR methods such as, for example, focus group discussions (FGDs) and individual-depth-interviews (IDIs) were used; techniques relied heavily on role plays.

D.4.2   Culturally-adapted Social Marketing (CASM)

The insight that CASOMAR provided formed the basis for designing the CASM strategies. These involved a multi-pronged approach: appropriate posters were placed in local bars, hairdressing saloons, kiosks; appropriate dramas, songs and poems were performed; information was channelled through schools and local organisations; training was offered to community health workers (CHWs) and traditional birth attendants (TBAs).

Efforts were made in the slum area to sensitise communities to the modes of transmission of HIV/AIDS/STDs, and to show that HIV/AIDS was a problem. The involvement of communities in the slum area was a major step in creating impact. Communities accepted that 'AIDS was a killer', and they began to accept AIDS orphans as their responsibility. From their own discussion and analysis, they identified project activities which were needed in the area. They formed pressure groups amongst themselves where they were able to identify sustainable income-generating projects like nursery schools, revolving funds and handicraft production.

The local communities acknowledge that the partner NGOs will not be working with them indefinitely, and are trying to arm themselves with the necessary ideas and experience to continue the work begun in Kibera. After seeing the community mobilisation and action, the Kenyan government provided the programme with a piece of land free of charge, which otherwise would have cost US $30,000.

D.5   CULTURALLY-APPROPRIATE OPTIONS

D.5.1   Home-based Care

Since the initiator and director of the programme had a professional nursing background, she was allowed by the Ministry of Health to run a regular clinic in Kibera for antenatal and post natal care. She also taught women the basics of primary health care, and especially how to take care of an AIDS patient at home in the absence of proper sanitary facilities. She taught basic counselling, and provided community training on the dangers posed by HIV/AIDS/STDs. Sometimes HIV/AIDS tests were provided free, and medical bills were waived for AIDS patients and orphans. From a 100 cases of STDs being seen weekly at the programme centre, there are now around 10 cases a week. This probably indicates changes in behaviour and health-seeking treatment.

Home Care

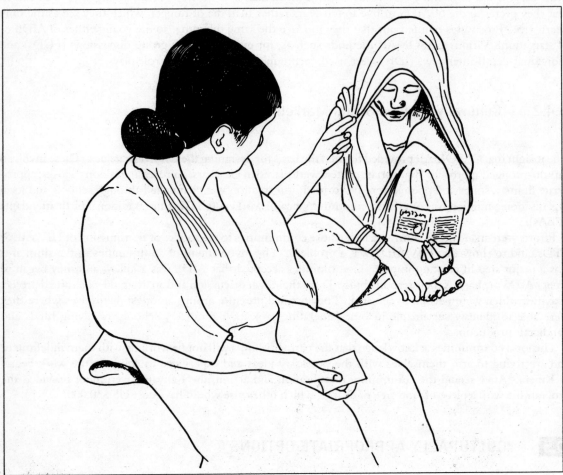

D.5.2   Action for AIDS Orphans

Since the centre began operating in 1993, more than 200,000 people have been reached, 50,000 have been treated which included 650 AIDS orphans. The latter are currently staying at the programme centre and going to the informal school built for them. The school teaches up to class four and has six teachers. They are not formally trained, but since the government recognises the value of the work being accomplished, it has changed its policy by agreeing to provide trained teachers, and also training the untrained teachers.

D.5.3   Use of Condoms

Members of the community living in the slum area are now accepting the use of condoms. All CASM activities emphasised the importance of using condoms during sexual intercourse. In line with donors' advice, the programme tried to levy a small charge of one Kenyan shilling per condom, the equivalent of about one US cent. Yet, the community could not afford to pay even this small amount. Their response was that they would have to do without condoms. It was then decided that condoms would be distributed free of charge. There are now 25 condom distribution points that together distribute 36,000 condoms a week. These free condoms are in great demand and are highly valued.

D.5.4   Teenage Forum

A weekly programme has been started for teenagers to create forums for them to discuss issues related to AIDS. Every week around 300 teenagers turn up for an hourly meeting.

D.6   NETWORKING INCREASES EFFECTIVENESS AND SUSTAINABILITY

The programme has established contact between the communities, the government services, and various NGOs working in the slum area, particularly those dealing with water and health services. Regular self-evaluation of the programme is carried out by programme staff, together with the communities they serve. Communities themselves are now seeing the impact of the programme on their local environment, their health, living conditions, and the impact of other NGOs in the area.

When the Ministry of Education came to the area to evaluate the effect of the informal school in the area, they interviewed parents (men and women), school teachers and schoolchildren. This alerted people about the importance of education. As a result, they divided themselves into six groups to help support education. One group has decided to make all the uniforms for the children, another group has decided to do voluntary carpentry work with the children, and another engaged in fishing has offered to give the children at least one meal every week. The Ministry of Education also wants to strengthen informal schools in the area, and has chosen the informal school started by the Kibera Self-help Programme as a pilot project to expand informal education in the whole country. The programme has also successfully negotiated with the government to allow pupils without school uniform to attend school. Earlier, this rule often prevented poor children from attending school. Government policy has now been changed to allow attendance without uniform. Also, children are to get free breakfast and lunch at school, and some help will be provided so that informal schools can get tables and chairs. The general approaches for programme networking and action adopted by the Kibera Self-help Programme have provided models for other NGOs in Kenya.

The programme has introduced training for small-scale business women, with credit made available for those who complete their training. These women were formerly vulnerable to prostitution due to financial insecurity. Prostitution, for many poor women, is not a profession but simply a temporary or long-term survival strategy resorted to when other strategies fail. It may also be temporarily adopted at certain life stages, in between more stable conjugal relationships.

D.7 CONSTRAINTS AND FURTHER CHALLENGES FOR THE KIBERA PROGRAMME

During the past five years, the programme has experienced various constraints, such as lack of personnel, lack of sustainability of some programme activities, lack of electricity (particularly to enable refrigeration of medicines), inadequate medicines for AIDS patients and for AIDS orphans. A vehicle is needed to help carry out programme activities, especially carrying the sick to hospitals, AIDS orphans to amusement parks and for making field trips. Communities have requested a delivery room within the existing clinic at the programme centre because they know that many women die during childbirth at home. The programme initiator hopes to see sustainable community activities developing, such as those begun by a group of community women, who have been trained and now run their own nursery school. They have also started a handicraft project to enable them to pay their house rents, buy a balanced diet, and access schools and medical care. It is hoped that the government will now help to build a hostel, provide better maternity care and roads. The expanding programme needs more staff and basic remuneration for them.

The Kibera programme is an outstanding example of the efficiency of CASM. Many cultural variables combine to complicate the existence and expansion of the programme. But, government support and development of a stronger and more financially sustainable base will probably ensure the future of the programme. The cultural and socio-economic context shifts continually as the number of potential consumers increases, HIV-infected individuals die, and new dynamic community actions are generated. The emerging experience of the programme is being marketed nationally and internationally as a practical and successful example of home-based care and related action for HIV/AIDS/STDs.

D.8 THE GROWTH OF SOCIAL MARKETING FOR HIV/AIDS/STDs

Culturally-appropriate social marketing in the field of HIV/AIDS has a special significance. Since 1987, when recognition began to grow that the world needed to brace itself against an impending pandemic, social marketing has been on the HIV/AIDS agenda. In the early days, it was used to construct potential user profiles of those target groups most at risk to, and affected by the pandemic. For example, high risk target groups such as homosexual men, prostitutes and commercial travellers were identified. Then, culturally appropriate strategies and practical approaches were developed at various sequential stages of the pandemic to meet the needs of the expanding categories of potential consumers.

Key cultural variables related to the HIV/AIDS pandemic are in many places closely related to poverty. For example, people who are poor usually have less access to health care, so they often come late for diagnosis (they are afraid to be tested), and are thus late for the treatment of the early signs and symptoms. They are less likely to get treatment for sexually transmitted diseases, and less likely to get and use condoms. HIV infection and AIDS contributes to household and individual impoverishment through job and income loss, rejection, and discrimination and stigmatisation against those affected by the virus. Families trying to cope with HIV and AIDS often feel marginalised. Both patients and their carers may find it difficult to talk about the problem with neighbours and friends, and may be reluctant to ask for help. The chronic nature and eventual fatal outcome, until a cure is found for the disease, also contributes to poverty.

The degree to which HIV/AIDS affects a poor household depends on the existing household income level—or poverty level—and where an HIV-infected household member/or members is/are situated on a scale ranging from initial infection to full-blown AIDS. For example, during a long asymptomatic phase normal occupation may be pursued. But, there can also be periods of relatively good health interspersed with bouts of serious illness. Where HIV transmission is sexual, it is common in developing countries to find that both spouses are ill at the same time, with the burden of care falling on the children, or a relative. Many cases of HIV are detected in a couple when a new-born child fails to thrive, or dies of an AIDS-related illness. Urban patients sometimes move back to rural areas to be looked after by relatives, and rural patients move to towns to take up trading when they can no longer farm. A household affected by HIV/AIDS often starts to become poorer by having to hire oxen (if they do not own them) for planting, which family members are too weak to do for themselves. They may have to hire expensive labour to do weeding. It is now believed that unless men assist women in labour tasks (which until recently were only performed by women) poverty, food insecurity and vulnerability will increase. For example, in some areas of Zambia, men have begun to acknowledge women's rights to have separate credit, fields and income, and are letting the women sell their own crops in the market. After the death of a breadwinner due to AIDS, the household sometimes splits apart. For example, in parts of central Africa, it is the custom for the dead husband's relatives to arrive after (or even before) his death to claim all household possessions—right down to the last cooking pot. Family members take unpaid leave from work to act as carers. Children take time off from school to take care of family members who are sick. The burden of home-care predictably falls on women. This means that women may have less time for agriculture.

D.8.1   Social Marketing of Appropriate Messages

In designing messages for HIV/AIDS/STDs, various key cultural variables have to be borne in mind. For example, many people are not aware that the body has an immune system. It is therefore difficult to explain to them that HIV infects and damages that system. It is hard for them to understand the concept of opportunistic infections, and why patients with different illnesses, such as diarrhoea, tuberculosis or shingles are all diagnosed as having AIDS. It is also hard to understand how a person who appears to be well could be an HIV carrier. While people of a higher educational level are more responsive to messages based on facts and figures, for those who are barely or non-literate, the approach is to build on their existing concepts of disease and family values. For example, in Kenya the slogan of 'zero grazing' was adopted. This is a concept used by cattle herdsmen to describe the practice of keeping a cow tied to a stake so that it only grazes in a single place and does not wander. In other places, proverbs or religious texts were used in a similar way. Humour is often used, and positive advice and images indicating what people CAN do are given. Local expressions and slang are used for words such as sexual intercourse, oral sex, anal intercourse, penis, semen, vagina. For example, in some parts of Africa condoms are referred to as 'gumboots' and 'raincoats'.

Radio can be used in various ways, such as interviews with local communities, panel discussions where health workers and others answer listener's questions, short spot announcements, magazine programmes with music and information, short dramas or AIDS education themes built into existing 'soap operas', and competitions where the audience is asked to send in correct answers. However, in many developing countries, television and newspapers are available only to a small minority of the population, often restricted to the high income section of the urban population. A disadvantage with both radio and television is that there are often restrictions on the freedom to discuss sexual matters on the mass media whereas it would be acceptable to discuss these in person.

D.9   CASOMAR AND CASM FOR SPECIFIC GROUPS AT PARTICULAR RISK TO HIV/AIDS/STDs

This section focuses on examples of people at particular risk to HIV/AIDS/STDs. These are migrant workers and refugees, and out-of-school and 'socially apart' (marginalised) youth.

D.9.1   Migrant Workers and Refugees

Every year, millions of migrants and refugees leave their homes in search of work, peace or just survival. All too often, they find that HIV infection is part of the bargain. In 1994, it was estimated that there were over 43 million displaced people globally—20 million of whom had fled their countries, and 23 million who were displaced within their own countries. 85 million men and women globally were estimated to be migrant workers. Both migrants and refugees face a wide range of problems and difficulties when it comes to HIV/AIDS/STDs. They are often blamed for 'bringing' HIV and AIDS with them into a country. Migrants and refugees are probably at greater risk of contracting HIV/AIDS/STDs than indigenous populations because they are disadvantaged in terms of information on HIV/AIDS/STDs. Illiteracy can often be a major problem, along with lack of culturally-appropriate education materials written in their own languages. Immigration laws can also have a devastating impact on HIV transmission in migrant communities by discouraging illegal immigrants from accessing public health programmes and forcing those with HIV and AIDS underground for fear of deportation. Jobs available to migrant workers are traditionally the ones which the local population is reluctant to take on—harsh, physically demanding work, often with increasing health and safety risks. In such bleak conditions it is hardly surprising that many men turn to drink, gambling, drugs or sex to make up for their daily frustrations. Sex is the only means that offers men, cut off from their surroundings, the pleasure of physical contact and affection— whether it is with prostitutes or other migrants. In some South African mines, senior miners took younger male workers as their 'mine wives' as far back as the turn of the century. For younger migrants and refugees, selling sex may be their only means of survival. They are often forced to sell at any price and are unable to insist that customers use a condom, even if they can afford them.

D.9.1.1   *CASM Strategies*

Appropriate CASM approaches have been very difficult to find within these complex settings. One successful example is where Dutch outreach workers distributed invitations to young Romanians (probably working as male prostitutes) to attend a meeting and promised to pay US $13 to those who turned up. Thirty did, and the meeting was very successful. The issues of HIV/AIDS/STDs were discussed with the help of an interpreter. The outreach workers gathered information on the living conditions of the Romanians and on their specific needs, which helped them produce effective and culturally relevant HIV/AIDS/STD information in Romanian.

D.9.2 Out-of-School and Socially Apart Youth

Another example of people at particular risk to HIV/AIDS/STDs are out-of-school youth. Millions of young people world-wide do not attend school. Some drop out of school because of poverty. Their families cannot afford school fees and/or the children must work to support the family income. Young women sometimes leave school to prepare for marriage, or are compelled to remain at home to perform domestic tasks. Also important in this context is the fact that certain ethnic groups are marginalised and discriminated against.

A majority of these children live in poor communities, often in female-headed households. Many such families have little or no access to basic social services. Increasing numbers of children also leave, or are driven from, their homes due to armed conflict or domestic violence and end up living on the streets. These young people have been described as being 'socially apart'. Often living in social and economic misery, such youth are at particular risk to HIV infection.

D.9.2.1 CASM Strategies

These strategies have included identifying individuals, who live near the marginalised youth concerned, to help sustain needed medical care (e.g., street vendors, dormitory supervisors, night porters at clinics, clergy members, sex workers) and provision of outreach services by health professionals directly in the settings of the youth e.g., worksites, transitory accommodations, shelters, correctional facilities. Specific guidelines and mapping techniques have been developed for and with the youth to ensure that they know where to go and with whom to speak when they need support or services. Free condoms are distributed through community-based clinics, NGOs, pharmacists, neighbourhood associations and youth clubs. Mass media has been used to sensitise the public to the plight of socially apart youth. The youth themselves have been involved in designing, pre- and post-testing educational resources made for them such as cartoon booklets. Using pictures from old magazines, they have constructed visual games and activity cards. Drama has proved to be an excellent tool to help young people deal with conflicts, mixed feelings, pains and joys surrounding the issues of sexuality and the risks of HIV/AIDS/STDs. The use of puppets in particular can help them express hidden feelings, worries, doubts and questions. Posters are hung up where meals are taken, videos are shown in shelters, workplaces and homes, games are played while visiting children in the streets, sexual health education using pictures is given during clinic visits. Those who work with out-of-school and socially apart youth have had to learn counselling skills, including dealing with sensitive topics like unwanted pregnancy and induced abortion. They help the youth to reflect on their feelings, experiences and needs. They also help them to identify practical options for action, and for behaviour change.

WHO, developed a particular 'narrative research' method in order to provide policy-makers and programme planners with a better understanding of how young people think and act. As greater attention is paid to young people's health and development, there is a corresponding increase in the demand for methods to collect information about their behaviour and views, which is essential to the development of appropriate action to meet their needs and help to solve their problems. Although a number of methods already exist for exploring young people's knowledge, attitudes and behaviour, they all have limitations. They tend to focus on single events rather than on the continuum and context of behaviour, and are usually generated from what adults believe to be relevant and significant to young people.

The narrative research method makes use of the most valuable resource we have in understanding patterns of young people—the young people themselves. It is designed to elucidate the most common patterns of social and sexual relationships which exist in a given society among young people as seen through their own eyes. It begins with a workshop for youth leaders between 18–25 years of age. They themselves develop a questionnaire identifying major events between puberty, marriage and childbearing. They then **create two adolescent characters, male and female, and role-play the first encounter between them.** A discussion around the last event portrayed leads to a group decision as to what event is likely to follow. They then role-play that event. The discussions and role plays continue until a full sexual and reproductive history has been developed. Each day the events are role-played and the subsequent discussions form the development of the questionnaire. The participants then return to their own communities with the questionnaires. After the questionnaires are completed, another workshop is held in which the storylines collected are analysed by the youth leaders using key cultural variables of gender, rurality, age and the like. They then discuss programme implications. This method has been used successfully in Africa, Latin America, Asia and Europe.

D.9.2.2   CASM in the School Setting

In 1994, WHO and UNESCO produced a three-part resource package (for curriculum planners, teachers and students) for school health education. This includes a variety of approaches to gathering information on student knowledge, attitudes and practices. There are basic illustrated questions and answers setting out why knowledge of HIV/AIDS/STDs is important, and how teachers can provide instructions for carrying out the learning activities. In the first part of the three-volume package there are a variety of materials (mostly single sheets designed for photocopying) relating to basic knowledge on HIV/AIDS/STDs. For example, short self-completion 'fun tests' and word-matching to pictures, true and false tests, self-assessment ('what is your risk?'), sheets on 'AIDs help, who, where?', a sheet to complete and identify how in various situations advice from the 'doctor's bag' can be useful. The second set of sheets deal with CASM for responsible behaviour e.g., delaying sex. These include 'reasons to say no' (using pictures and a self-scoring system), guidelines with a checklist for help to delay sex (writing in boxes the things that the learner would find easy to do, and those difficult to do,) how to show affection without sex, assessment of assertiveness, construction of assertive messages, how to respond to persuasion (e.g., writing captions on pictures) agree/disagree about gender relationships and sex, and dealing with threats and violence. Another set of sheets deals with 'responsible behaviour: protected sex'. It includes activities and materials relating to use of condoms, a demonstration on how to say no to unprotected sex. Self-assessment and pictures are extensively used in the package. The last set of sheets is 'care and support' and deals with discrimination, community responses, importance of compassion, how to give care, how to keep safe, support for responsible behaviour. Statement completion, stories and answers, and bubble captions are the methods used.

This resource package includes a collection of imaginative CASM techniques and can be obtained from WHO/UNESCO offices.

D.9.3   CASM in the Workplace

CASM methods and techniques have also been used in the workplace. For example, commercial farm owners in Zimbabwe are promoting AIDS prevention activities that have the support of employees and their families. Many workers live with their families in settlements owned by agricultural or mining companies. These include large commercial farms in Zimbabwe, sugar, tobacco and tea plantations in Tanzania and India, and mines in Brazil and Botswana. Management usually provides basic housing, health care and education. In Zimbabwe, the Commercial Farmers Union (CFU), representing over 4,500 farm owners and managers, has been developing HIV prevention programmes for farm workers since 1986. Once they are familiar with the issues, volunteer co-ordinators from branch associations of the CFU begin discussions first with village leaders, and then the wider community. Condoms, paid for by the farm owners, are available from the village health worker, or farm clerk, from farm shops, with the pay packet (with the agreement of workers) and also from selected individuals. AIDS committees are set up at village level, involving local men and women. There is now greater demand for condoms and fewer cases of STDs. Single women are turning from selling sex to seeking paid farm work. There is now considerable community pride that the challenge has been faced. AIDS is treated like any other disease, and the degree of stigma has been reduced.

In India, an AIDS research foundation is being financed by local companies to train key employees. The most difficult part of developing a workplace programme and policy was found to be in persuading company directors to accept responsibilities towards their employees. They were found to be more willing to listen if met 'on their own turf' such as through social clubs, and civic organisations like the Rotary Club. A specific campaign is developed for each company. Most employers agree to the distribution of condoms at the workplace, through medical dispensaries and through individual workers selling condoms. For small businesses, interventions were designed not only for the factory workers and sales representatives, but also for the small trucking ventures and drivers who buy the tyres. Condoms are sold in roadside stalls, and to women selling sex to both drivers and salesmen. The foundation was investigating the possibility of financing the duplication of a cassette tape of songs on safe behaviour, along with tyre advertisements which could be played in the teashops along the road.

D.9.3.1   Empowerment Training

Another type of CASM in the workplace involved the half kilometre area of Bangkok known as 'Patpong' where at least 400 women work on any one night. From the 1980s onwards, with tourism as a major income earner in Thailand, Patpong became a major sex entertainment centre. Most of the women, originally from poor drought stricken areas, were illiterate. In 1986 the 'empowerment training' programme opened with ten students in one bar. By 1989 there were 385 students, including dancers, waitresses, shop clerks, street vendors, bar tenders, male prostitutes and tourist guides. The six week training included reading, writing and drama. The women scripted their own stories. A community newspaper was produced, providing a means for 'voiceless' people to communicate their ideas and opinions. There was a documentation centre for women's studies. 'Empowerment training' offered health education, bar visits, counselling and workshops relating to media issues and materials. A leaflet and booklet on AIDS was distributed, and a mobile exhibition launched. Empowerment action involved encouraging women to take leadership roles in educating their friends, persuading customers to use condoms, obtaining co-operation of managers and *mamasans*, and educating customers, press and media about safer sex and condoms.

D.10   CASM AND HOMECARE

Innovative homecare programmes, such as the Kibera self-help scheme, provide a variety of services to people with HIV infection and their families; these have been developing in Africa from 1987. They reflect different health, cultural and philosophical concepts. A six-country study in 1991 looked at programmes which had been in operation for around two years. These included government, non-government, community-initiated, rural, urban, hospital-based, non-hospital-based programmes and programmes with various religious affiliations. Basic information was collected through interviews with key informants, group interviews with health staff, interviews with patients and their families, on-site observations, and collection of additional documentary material.

Culturally-appropriate services provided in these homecare programmes included hospital care, where available, for those requiring specialised care (e.g., those with severe weight loss, anaemia, tuberculosis). Programmes usually have clinics for adults and children with HIV and AIDS, involving medical care, clinical diagnosis, symptomatic treatment, free drugs, including herbal remedies, nursing care, counselling and material support. Counsellors trained for HIV/AIDS may visit HIV-positive patients in the wards to arrange for follow-up and homecare. Transportation is often a problem for the poorest patients. Home-based care may be carried out by mobile teams, visiting one family every 2–3 months, community counselling on main modes of HIV transmission, training of AIDS health promotion officers, and community action for HIV/AIDS/STD prevention and control. Also, management training seminars for health care providers and collaborators.

For patients living near health facilities, home visits take place by health care providers. A drop-in time is provided for clients who want counselling or information. In some cases this is linked to material assistance consisting of food supplement, soap, sheets, used clothing, school fees and the like. There may be a day-room where HIV-positive persons and their families can meet in a safe and supportive atmosphere. There may be opportunities for income-generating activities such as tailoring, mat-making, and sewing bed sheets and school uniforms. A day-room may offer relaxation classes and spiritual guidance. A pastoral care and counselling programme may take place in secondary schools aimed at reinforcing safe sex behaviour or bringing about behaviour change.

Advantages of homecare include continuity of treatment, decrease in demand for hospital beds, reduction of fear, prejudice and stigma. The main consequences of AIDS on family life include severe poverty, lack of food, rejection and isolation, eviction from home due to non-payment of rent. Many parents with AIDS are concerned not so much about dying, but about the future of their children. Grandmothers may be left to care for many orphans, especially in some areas where up to 50 per cent of the population is affected by AIDS. Culturally-appropriate options developed include programmes to help teach grandmothers how to farm and how to deal with house repairs.

D.11   WORLD-WIDE USAGE OF CASM

Hundreds and even thousands of AIDS awareness campaigns have been put into operation around the world. There is also an annual 'AIDS Day' each year when the attention of the world is drawn to a particular aspect of AIDS. Early in the pandemic it was realised that by itself information increases knowledge, but does not change behaviour. AIDS educators have to understand and confront people's fears, and make sure that the source of AIDs information can be trusted. To educate people about AIDS it was first necessary to overcome denial. AIDS information had to take account of actual sexual behaviour. Religion and culture were powerful in shaping attitudes to HIV/AIDS/STDs. AIDS education directed towards women had to take account of their social and cultural situations.

Many countries launched multi-media campaigns using television, advertising posters, pop music, radio programmes, demonstrations (e.g., proper use of condoms), children's stories, cartoon books, TV soap series. Depending on the prevailing culture and literacy levels these have, in varying degrees, achieved their objectives.

In **Zaire** in the late 1980s, one of the country's best known singers recorded an album with the title 'Watch Out for AIDS'. The music spread to Paris, London and New York, indicating the international nature of pop music.

In **Mexico** a pioneering youth movement with 26,000 members, has used glove puppets to spread the message about AIDS. At the cross-roads between two wide, dusty streets, groups of adults and children are often seen watching these puppet shows. They represents the story of community life using a variety of characters—a single mother, a young street child, a homosexual man, a factory worker. The story is not just for entertainment, it clearly shows the dangers of having unprotected sex with many partners.

In **Chile** an 'AIDS game' was developed. When they started talking about AIDS they realised that they had no teaching materials to share knowledge with people in a participatory way. So, in 1989, they developed a board game called **Learning About AIDS**. The game is based on the local people's experiences; it provides basic information on HIV/AIDS; encourages discussion about beliefs and myths about AIDS; provides opportunities for open exchange of opinions, and views about sexuality and AIDS; promotes awareness of how AIDs affects the community and the need for HIV prevention. The game uses two sets of cards: 72 'everyone's task' cards with questions on HIV transmission and prevention, and 35 'community cards' describing possible situations in the community where problems and issues about HIV and AIDS could arise. The issues are discussed in a booklet which accompanies the game. It is essential to have a skilled game facilitator who is aware of the issues that arise when talking about HIV and sexual health. People play the game in pairs using a dice. Each player in turn moves their counter forward the number of squares on the board shown on the dice. If the counter lands on a square marked with a number the person picks up a card and answers it. When a counter lands on a 'community' card square the whole group discuss the issue. These cards do not have 'right' or 'wrong' answers. The game was designed with a group of people involved in education or living with AIDS, and is based on real life experiences. Each group which uses the game can change it for local use. One group made a large-scale version on a football pitch, built life-size models of the community buildings and made a giant dice. The game enables players to obtain useful information, access services and change social attitudes to enable every individual to develop their own sexuality healthily and safely.

In **East Asia**, through a local NGO in Timor, an HIV/AIDS/STD prevention programme carried out a study in 12 villages to identify the main causes of HIV transmission. The team was made up of NGO staff, two retired nurses, a religious leader and several village health workers. All were known and respected by local people. Information was gathered through in-depth interviews and focus group discussions with traditional healers, religious leaders and young people. The interviews usually started with a conversation about general health in the community. Once the issue of sexual health had been mentioned, staff explained the aim of the study and people were invited to participate. It was emphasised that anything they said would be anonymous. Discussions were usually held in small single-gender groups. People were very open provided that the setting was relaxed and informal. One practice that could lead to HIV/STD transmission was found to be the custom of male circumcision at puberty. After the circumcision has been done by traditional practitioners, young men are required to have sexual intercourse with 2–4 different women. People also discussed issues such as multiple sex partners, abortion, teenage pregnancy, family planning including access to condoms, and young people leaving the area. Methods included 'body mapping' where participants were asked to draw their own genitals. There was usually much laughter at the beginning of this approach, but after a while most participants started to draw seriously. After the exercise participants usually spoke more openly about sexuality. Role-plays were also used. The key successes of the programme have been openness about sexuality, a relaxed atmosphere, involvement of all groups in the community, and the avoidance of moralising. On a few occasions single-gender sessions were held to encourage women to speak up. The 11 study findings were presented to officials at the district level, who agreed to support an HIV/STD education programme. The programme began to co-operate with the health service, churches, schools and government.

D.12 CONCLUSION

These case materials have thrown into relief the need for cultural sensitivity in trying to reduce the danger HIV/AIDS/STD presents to present and future generations. As can be seen, there exists already a wealth of experience in the use of CASM in the context of HIV/AIDS/STD. This clearly indicates the important part CASM can play not only in raising public awareness of the threat HIV/AIDS/STD poses to humanity but, even more importantly in reducing the spread of these killer diseases.

D.13 RECOMMENDED READING

Castle, C. and **A. Filgueras** (1993). *Resource Pack on Sexual Health and Aids Prevention for Socially Apart Youth-Hand in Hand Network*, AHRTAG and SOS Crianca, Brazil.

Feuerstein, M.T. and **H. Lovel** (1989). 'Community Responses to Aids' Special Issue of the *Community Development Journal*, Volume 24, Number 3.

Feuerstein, M.T. (1997). *Health and Poverty*, Macmillan, London.

Covarrubias, S. (1995). 'AIDS, Everyone's Task', *Aids Action Issue* 30, September–November, pp. 6–7.

Fraser-Mackenzie (1992). 'Caring Companies?', *Aids Action Issue* 18, p. 5.

Hampton, J. and **G.A. Williams** (1990). Living Positively With Aids: The Aids Support Organization (TASO) Uganda, MS. (Available from TALC).

Hubley, J. (1990). *The Aids Handbook: A Guide to the Understanding of Aids and HIV*, Macmillan, London.

Hughes, H. (1989). 'A Day in the Life of Gente Joven' in *Aids Action Issue* 6. International Planned Parenthood Federation (IPPF) (1988). *Talking AIDS: A Guide for Community Work*, IPPF, London.

Hulewicz, J.M. and **Panos** (1994). 'AIDS Knows No Borders', *Worldaids*, September, pp. 6–10.

Owiti, A. (1996). 'Report on Kibera Community Self Help Programme, Nairobi, Kenya' for the Third International Conference on Evaluation of Social Development, 4–8 November, Netherlands, MS.

Panos (1988). *Aids and The Third World—Panos Dossier*, Panos Institute with the Norwegian Red Cross, London, Oslo.

Sundararaman, S. (1992). 'Prevention: Who Pays?', *Aids Action Issue* 18, p. 5.

WHO (1991) 'Report of the World Health Organization/Commonwealth Secretariat Regional Workshop on HIV/Aids Community-based Care and Control'. Entebbe, (Uganda) October.

——— (1991). *Living With Aids in the Community—A Book To Help People Make the Best of Life*, written and produced in the Republic of Uganda, WHO/GPA/IDS/HCS/92.1, revised by WHO and UNICEF 1992.

——— (1991). *Review of Six HIV/Aids Home Care Programmes in Uganda and Zambia*, GPA/IDS/HCS/91.3, MS.

——— (1993). 'Adolescent Sexual Behaviour and Reproductive Health: From Research to Action'. Report of a Joint Meeting Dakar, Senegal April 1993, WHO/ADH/93.5.

——— (1995). 'Manual of Group Interview Techniques to Assess the Needs of People With AIDS' WHO/GPA/TCO/HCS/95.2.

WHO/UNESCO (1994). *School Health Education to Prevent AIDS and STD* (A Resource Package for curriculum planners,: Teacher's Guide, Students activities, and Handbook for curriculum planners), WHO/GPA/TCO/PRV/94.6a.

Case Study E

A UK Drugs Information Study Focusing on Children Aged 9–10[1]

Hermione Lovel

ABSTRACT

This project took seven months and followed established social marketing strategies. It began with a detailed review and analysis of relevant literature. This helped to design the focus and research methodology of the subsequent primary data collection. The research findings formed the basis for developing and piloting the fun, iridescent, amusing, thought provoking and participatory (add your own pictures and comments) leaflets, which were pilot tested.

E.1 BASIC SOCIAL MARKETING (SM) PRINCIPLES AND HOW THEY WERE APPLIED IN THIS PROJECT

E.1.1 Identifying Need, Entering a People's World and Understanding their Perspective of Life

The key philosophy in social marketing is based on the principle of learning all there is to know about the consumer and developing initiatives **with** rather than **for** the consumer.

E.1.2 Consumer Orientation and Consumer-led Activities

These are the essential pre-conditions of commercial marketing success. To understand and empathise with the target audience enquiry, which will illuminate how people **think** and **feel** about things, is

---

[1] This material is drawn from the report by Baker and Caraher, 1995 (see E.7).

needed. Thus, if effective health communication is to be produced, it is necessary to understand and empathise with the perceptions, motivations, behaviour and above all the needs of the consumer. Methods are needed which explore perceptions and attitudes, which then shape the development of the product. Methods which will gauge emotional responses that can be used to pilot media prototypes are also needed.

E.1.3   Qualitative Research Methods

These methods, which are widely used in market research, have been found to be most effective in eliciting information about the perceptions, motivations and needs of children aged 9–10. The aim was to start from the mindset of the child. This does not mean that an acceptance of what children believe or how they behave is required, but starting with this insight and understanding helps to make sense of their responses.

E.1.4   Target Segmentation

Done by grouping people who have similarities such as age, gender and social class, target segmentation is a means to effectively identify people's needs. Market segmentation results in a number of target groups, each of which is socially fairly homogenous. The specification of a well defined and homogenous audience can be the key to a successful programme.

E.1.4.1   *Primary Target Group: School Children Aged 9–10*

In the course of development of a drugs resource in the UK, it was realised that an audience defined by age (9–10 year old children) was not necessarily a homogenous group. Other studies of drugs and young people found that drugs education or prevention programmes need to take account of individual differences in the level of drug use and the stage of use (non-starter to regular). Thus it is suggested that any such programme needs to take account of five stages in the acquisition of a drug use habit:

* Pre-contemplation (never considered using a drug).
* Contemplation (considered using a drug).
* Preparation (preparing to try a drug).
* Action (experimental drug use).
* Maintenance (regular drug use).

However, in the context of the project discussed here, it was realised that it would be difficult to find out or to judge drug use behaviour among 9–10 year olds. Attempting to divide them into such groups might also cause awkwardness, ethical difficulties and be counter-productive to the rest of the project. It was agreed instead that the resource should be adaptable enough to take account of the different stages at which the children might be.

In this project, children were identified as the primary audience and parents, teachers and other significant adults as the secondary audience.

E.1.4.2   Secondary Target Group: Parents and Teachers

The key question in social marketing is not just 'who is the resource intended for?' but also 'who does it need to be acceptable to?' Again the drugs education literature was a help in defining the importance of this social marketing concept of secondary audiences. It was already recognised that the involvement and support of parents is an important factor in ensuring the effectiveness of any messages about drugs education. Also if schools and parents convey radically different messages to children, children will reject one or the other or both sets of messages.

E.1.5   Exchange Theory

Barter, purchases, marketing, all involve exchange between marketer and consumer. In 'ordinary' marketing, consumers who buy something of a particular brand perceive that they have gained quality, value for money, or social status. In social marketing the exchange is seen as **voluntary** and **mutually beneficial.** The perceived gain in social marketing is just as important as in other marketing fields. Thus enquiry is always needed to unearth values and appreciation that can then be used to include perceived gain in the prototypes developed. Secondary data search on drugs education for 9–10 year olds indicated that there was very little information available to identify what this target group might appreciate in a drugs education resource. Most drugs education and prevention research has focused on teenagers. However, a few studies and one large piece of research on 2,000 children aged 4–11 were found.

E.1.6   Lessons Learnt from the Secondary Data Survey

It has been argued that educating children about drugs is inappropriate, unnecessary and may even increase drug use. However, a Dublin study has shown that 60 per cent of the children surveyed had been offered drugs before they reached 15 years of age and drugs experimentation was most likely between the ages of 10 and 14. Other studies showed similar findings and also suggested that taking drugs increases markedly after age 15. These surveys suggested that drugs education may not be inappropriate for 9–10 year olds as it can prepare them for an imminent time when drugs may be offered to them or they may see them in use.

E.1.6.1   The Socio-cultural Setting of 9–10 Year Olds

The age of 9–10 is a period of great transition for children in the UK. They are often concerned about the transition from primary to secondary school at age 11. There may be fears of bullying, fears of moving to a bigger school with a larger and more formal classroom environment. The change in school may be marked by various *rites de passage* associated with a need to belong or to rebel. It was recognised that drugs education which starts at a time of crisis (e.g., when drugs are present in school) has missed the opportunity of preparing children in advance to deal with such a crisis if it arises.

E.1.6.2   The Meaning of 'Drugs Education' for Young People
Aged 9–10 and how they Use Information

A range of meanings were found from scare tactics, skills to encourage safer drug use, and provision of information. However scare tactics in education are now recognised as ineffective and misleading. It is also a false assumption that children use information as knowledge and that this is then a key factor to influence their attitudes and in turn their behaviour. While accurate information is essential, the knowledge is used in a social context which influences how the information is used. A young person who belongs to a social circle that is engaged in drug use may face a different set of choices from one who is not. Children may also hold contradictory views on drug taking, agreeing that people who take them 'are stupid' but also experimenting with drugs themselves.

Earlier drugs education leaflets assumed that children act rationally on information, however, it is now widely recognised that children may view the use of drugs as a positive alternative. The risk that taking drugs offers may be attractive to some children. Risks may also be downplayed and the benefits of drugs exaggerated to make the risks seem worthwhile. Children and adolescents may, because of their experience (or lack of it), assume that they are not likely to be in any danger. Risk taking is part of adolescence.

Overall it seemed from the literature that drugs information material perceived as unrealistic, impersonal, didactic, or judgmental was likely to be rejected. What was needed was sophisticated information on drugs which would both inform and challenge them in their decision-making.

E.1.6.3   The Need for Skill Development

A number of studies have begun to appreciate the need to develop skills in children in relation to drugs. But it is recognised merely listing coping strategies without developing critical consciousness and self-improvement is of no use. Self esteem is also associated with positive coping behaviours, provided that the skills have also been learnt. The social context always affects behaviour in using new skills. The need for personal support (by a motivator or facilitator) is known to encourage maintenance of preventive behaviours.

E.1.7   Designing for Children

Millions of pounds are spent on quality advertising for toys, sweets and entertainment for children. Any educational initiative will be in competition with such media. In addition, it is recognised that design for children should neither underestimate or undermine its audience; it needs to be in tune with, mediate and respect a child's wants. For a children-focused advertisement to reach its objectives it must convey that the product lets the child enjoy the experience of allowing participation; it must also highlight that it poses a challenge. Professional designers need to be involved to interpret children's needs and then to conduct children-led evaluation. It is important to listen to children, interpret their needs, and respect their wisdom.

E.2   THE RESEARCH

The lessons learnt from the literature review formed the basis for designing a strategy to develop the drugs information resource for children aged 9–10. The target area chosen was of manageable size with a socio-economic mix where the local drugs prevention unit already had good contacts with schools. Schools were concerned about possible parental objections to 'drugs research' so a consent form for parents and clear briefings for head teachers and class teachers were provided. Working through the local drugs prevention team made these issues easier to negotiate with the schools. The project was conducted in three stages:

    I. **The Listening Stage**
   II. **The Interpreting Stage**
  III. **The Piloting Stage**

The relationship between the researchers and the participants differed in the different stages.

E.3   RESEARCH AT THE LISTENING STAGE

E.3.1   Children, the Primary Audience

With children as the primary audience, the aim was to find out what the children spent their time thinking about, what they enjoyed doing, their concerns, fears and aspirations, who they perceived as authority figures and why and how much control they thought they would have in situations they feared. The transition from primary to secondary school was the specific context chosen for the focus of the questions.

E.3.1.1   *Draw and Write Techniques*

These techniques, which have a long history in health related research, to identify feelings about events, current knowledge and concerns, were used. The focus was not on how many children were using drugs but on children's perceptions of drug use and messages about drugs. The method enables interaction with children. The research methodology was based on co-operative enquiry

E.3.1.2   *The Self-portrait Exercise*

The researcher explained to the children that the aim was to find out how young people feel about going to secondary school. The children, were asked to work in pairs and trace out their head and shoulders on the wall. Then they were asked to work individually and to draw and/or write seven thought bubbles:

* Some things you like dreaming about.
* Some things you feel strongly about.
* Some things you like doing best.
* Your favourite possessions.
* Some dangers you think you might face in secondary school.
* Some things you would like to take to secondary school.
* How you might deal with those dangers.

The exercise took about two hours. Children could use words, pictures or both. They would explain drawings to the researcher when asked. There was no mention of drugs at this stage.

The session closed with children summarising the dangers raised, along with ideas on ways of dealing with the dangers. The researcher identified inventive proposals but did not pass judgement. 126 children participated in the exercise, which was enjoyed by all involved. The responses to each of the seven questions were then grouped into topics for analysis with a view to the marketing of a drugs education resource.

Schoolchildren Responding to Teacher

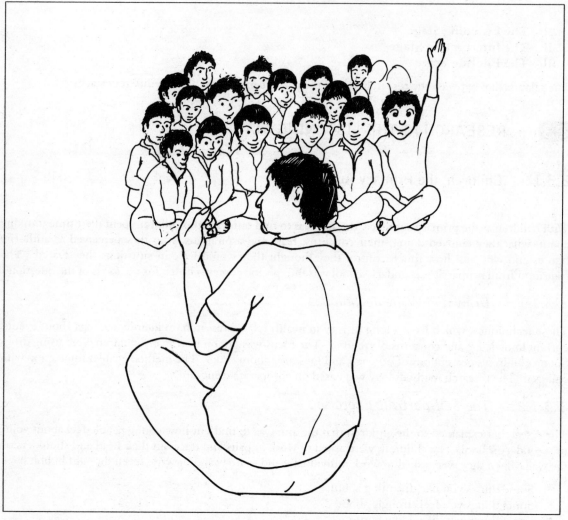

* **Dreams** were mostly self-centred. The world seemed full of opportunity and wealth. 'It was concluded that the drugs education resource should encourage the high aspirations and high self-confidence of the children. It could do this by encouraging and supporting each child's own decision-making ability in a non-didactic way, reaffirming the conclusions of the literature reviews.
* **Issues important to children** were affected by the topics discussed in recent school lessons (e.g., racism, drugs and pollution) but their wide-ranging responses implied that these issues were just the same real to them.
* **On what children like best doing** there were clear preferences for television, fast food and computers. This suggested that the drugs education needed to reflect the up-to-the-minute style

Schoolchildren Participating in the UK Drugs Information Study

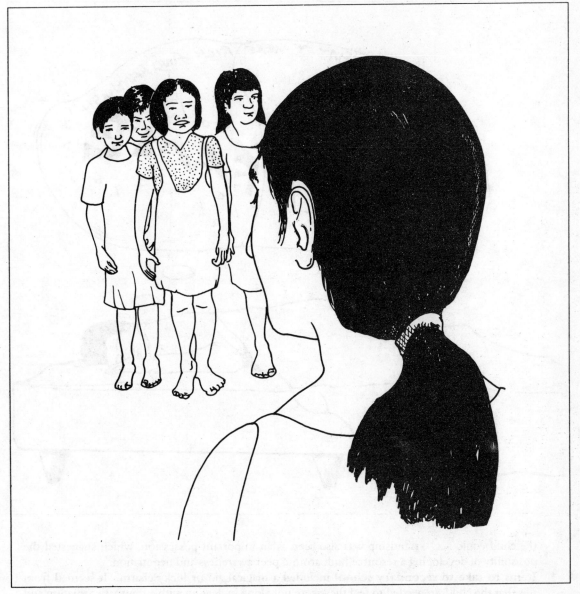

of commercial media if it was to be perceived as worthwhile. The preference shown for creative activities highlighted the need for some kind of activity that could encourage such creativity.

★ **Favourite possessions** were often interpreted as family, pets or private space (e.g., their bedroom). This suggested the resource material might somehow provide an individual secret area in which

What Children Dream About

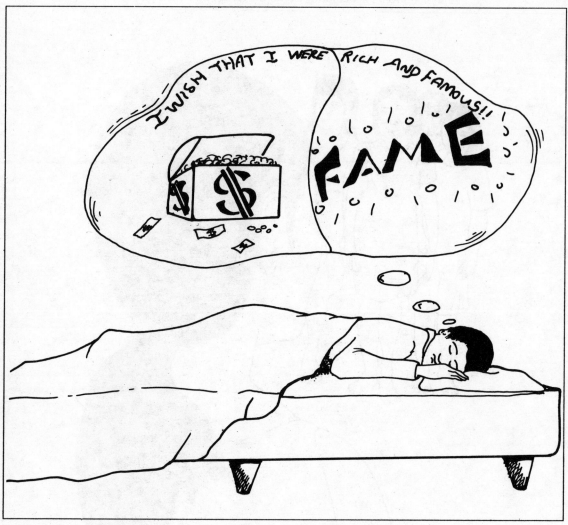

the child could act. Friendship was also seen as an important possession, which suggested the possibility of developing a resource built around peer awareness and negotiation.

* **Items to take to secondary school** included a magical aid or lucky charm. It seemed from this that the children needed to feel they were not alone in dealing with a traumatic situation and making their choices (so the final version frequently refers to 'your mate' (friend).

* **Dangers perceived** were the same for most respondents: i.e., bullying, smoking, drugs, violence and crime. Smoking and drugs were mentioned by 40 per cent of the 126 children. Some thought

they would be bullied into taking drugs, or that drugs were an unavoidable danger because of the temptation or that everyone was taking them. The implications for the drugs education was that there should be emphasis on individual choice.

★ **Dealing with the dangers:** Most children (55 per cent) said they would do so by going to a responsible adult (teachers, parents, police and people they trusted) and 5 per cent would want to fight back. From this it was decided it would be helpful to encourage children to see themselves and their peers as allies.

E.3.2   Parents/Governors, Teachers/School Nurses, and Head Teachers, the Secondary Audience

One to one interviews were used with two parents, one deputy principal teacher, four primary teachers and two school nurses. The national curriculum was also examined. The aim was to find out

- Whether and to what extent drugs was an issue.
- How the use of drugs was perceived.
- Their perceived roles in relation to drugs education.
- Their existing contact with drugs education.

Parents seemed taken aback and surprised, having thought that there was little danger in schools. The deputy head thought that there was already information in school amongst the children 'but probably picked up in the wrong circumstances'. The primary teachers said primary schools should be involved, and the school nurses felt that it should be part of personal and social education (PSE). From the curriculum examination it was apparent that the material needed to be flexible to fit into either a science curriculum or PSE.

E.4   RESEARCH AT THE INTERPRETATION STAGE

From the findings of Stage 1 some key design elements were targeted. These included a **'Me Box'** (that children could construct and put things into).

Another focus was to enable children to identify different options and judge each others choices. Producing a DIY (do it yourself) booklet, flat-packed so that children could construct it themselves, helped the activity to be creative, challenging and to lead to success and self esteem when done. The booklet was designed to be light-hearted and off-beat, with bright spot colours and unusual illustrations. The hand drawn style of lettering and shapes of numbers contributed to the off-beat style.

The small size was designed to enhance a feeling of 'ownership' with space on the spine, front and rear on which the children could write or draw to personalise the booklet. The inside back cover was designed for evaluation.

E.5   RESEARCH AT THE PILOTING STAGE

E.5.1   Piloting with the Children

Objectives set for the piloting stage of the booklet were that each child should:

- Feel a sense of ownership of their booklet and personal space.
- Understand the concept of drugs.
- Feel comfortable with their chosen mode of expression, i.e., drawing, writing or both.
- Consider the options available to them in potential drug-taking situations.
- Make a choice from these options.
- Discuss and negotiate with their peers.
- Think sequentially and consider consequences of their initial choice.
- Enjoy the exercise.
- Feel challenged by the experience.

133 children, from 5 of the 6 participating schools were involved. The classes were told that they were needed to help with making the booklets; each would make her/his own and the researcher would take them away for analysis and return them to each child. They were told that this was not a 'test' and there were no right or wrong answers.

Nearly every child personalised her/his book and took pride and effort in doing this. This clearly indicated a sense of ownership, including 'keep out' messages added to the front! Again, nearly all children completed the page listing drugs on the inside front cover. Most children expressed themselves in words and seemingly were happy in this medium although one wrote 'drawing is hard'.

Writing a **range** of options 'if you saw your mate taking drugs' was also done by most children. A number of children showed that they enjoyed the exercise. It gave them an opportunity to be creative and imaginative.

Ninety per cent of children then made a **choice** of one of the options, although not all realised that one column was for themselves and the other for their friend.

Discussion did occur with a friend, including disagreement.

Sequential thinking (what would happen next) was shown by most (81 per cent) indicating most realised the consequences of their actions.

The exercise seemed enjoyable to students and teachers alike. Some (11 per cent) found the making of booklets difficult suggesting that the exercise was a challenge.

E.5.2   Piloting with Parents and Teachers

A focus group was held with 18 **parents of children** between 5–14 years old. They were asked:

- What would you think if your child brought this booklet home from school?
- What do you think about the fact that this booklet contains no information?
- What would you think if your child brought this booklet home to do at home rather than at school?

In general parents responded favourably, although some wanted to talk about what other information about drugs would be available through the school. Some said clearly they would prefer drugs (and sex) education to take place at home.

The five teachers of the classes visited at the pilot stage were interviewed. The questions put to them were:

- What do you think of the booklet as a drugs education resource?
- What do you think about the fact that this booklet contains no information?
- Would you feel able to use this resource within the curriculum?

All found the booklet interesting and useful.

The piloting suggested the need for a number of changes in the drugs education resource: folding instructions needed to be made easier, the double layer of tick boxes was to be modified and the two part 'personal information' and 'what would you do if you were offered drugs?' might be put on two separate sheets.

A comparison was also made with a draft computer programme. The computer had 'appeal' but the booklet created more ownership. The booklet was also easier to use in a classroom with desks or tables, whereas the computer programme required individual computer access if 'ownership' of responses and the computer programme was to be achieved.

E.6 CONCLUSION

The perceptions, motivations, behaviour and needs of the primary and secondary audiences were elicited in three stages by means of a culturally-appropriate qualitative research, the findings of which led to the development of innovative and effective drugs education resource materials. This case study throws into relief the necessity to investigate and understand the mindset not only of the primary but also the secondary target. This is frequently overlooked in projects that aim to effect socially desirable behavioural changes.

E.7 RECOMMENDED READING

Advisory Council on the Misuse of Drugs (ACMD) (1993). *Drug Education in School: The Need for New Impetus*, HMSO, London.

Ajzen, I. and **M. Fishbein** (1980). *Understanding Attitudes and Predicting Social Behaviour*, Prentice Hall, Englewood NJ.

Baker, H. and **M. Caraher** (1995). *Do it yourself: the process of developing a drugs information resource for children*. UK Central Drugs Prevention Unit. Home Office Drugs Prevention Initiative Paper 6.

Coles, R. (1986). *The Political Life of Children*, Houghton Muflin, Boston.

Dorn, N. (1984). *Drugs in Health Education: Trends and Issues*, ISDD, London.

Dorn, N. and **K. Murji** (1992). *Drug Prevention: A Review of the English Language Literature*, Research Monograph 5.ISDD, London.

Hastings, G.B. and **A. Haywood** (1991). 'Social Marketing and communication in health promotion' *Health Promotion International* 6(2), pp. 135–45.

Heller, S. and **S. Guarnaccia** (1994). *Designing for Children*, Watson-Guptill Publications, New York.

Kotler, P. and **G. Zaltman** (1971). 'Social Marketing: An approach to planned social change' *Journal of Marketing* 43, pp. 29–36.

Patton, M.Q. (1987). *Creative Evaluation*, Sage Publications, California.

Pridmore, P. (1994). 'Three approaches to participative enquiry', in N.K. Denzin and Y. Lincoln (eds), *Handbook of Qualitative Research*, Sage Publications, California.

Starr, C. (1969). 'Social Benefit versus technological risk' *Science* 165, pp. 1232–38.

Tobler, N.S. (1986). 'Meta Analysis of 143 adolescent drug prevention programmes' *Journal of Drug Issues* 16(4), pp. 537–38.

Tones, K. and **S. Tilford** (1994). *Health Education Effectiveness, Efficiency and Equity*, Chapman Hall, London.

Wallack, L.M. (1981). 'Mass media campaigns: The odds against finding behaviour change' *Health Education Quarterly* 8, 209–60.

Werch, C.E. and **C. Di Clemente** (1994). 'A multi-component stage model for matching drug prevention strategies and messages to youth—stage of use' *Health Education Research* 9(1), pp. 37–46.

Case Study F

AIDPLUS (INDIA) Raises Funds

Ajit Mani and Susan Thomas

F.1   INTRODUCTION

This case illustrates how culturally-adapted social marketing research (CASOMAR) and culturally-adapted social marketing (CASM) were applied by the field director of a British charity in India. Although all names mentioned in this case are fictitious, it is based on a real-life situation.

F.1.1   Mark Collet's Mission

Mark Collet was the field director of AIDPLUS (INDIA) Society, one of the oldest and most respected international charities working in India. Collet himself came from a line of 'old India hands' and could trace his ancestry in India back to the times of the East India company. Several years of patient research on his family tree had shown that one of his ancestors, Joseph Collet, had been the president of Fort St. George in Madras, and had had the singular honour of consolidating East India Company's power on the Coromandel Coast under the famous 1717 Imperial *farman*, which historians of the British Empire have called the Magna Carta of India.

    Mark Collet's father was a missionary who had worked for 32 years in Bengal. Collet himself had spent the early years of his life growing up in the mission compound at Bolangir (in what is now the state of Orissa), in the company of *ayahs*, (nannies) and Indian friends. He spoke Oriya, Bengali and Hindi and loved India. He had taken this assignment because AIDPLUS INTERNATIONAL wanted AIDPLUS (INDIA) to achieve a measure of autonomy and raise its own funds in India.

    India was coming out of its economic isolation by the 1980s, and there was a flourishing, Westernised middle class with an income large enough to spend on luxuries and spare a bit for charity. Collet had been given a *carte blanche* to initiate a market research study and come up with a proposal to start fund-raising in India for AIDPLUS (INDIA).

F.1.2   AIDPLUS (INDIA)

AIDPLUS had seven field offices in India. They were located in Kanpur, Mumbai, Ahmedabad, Patna, Chennai, Bhubaneshwar, and Calcutta. The work of AIDPLUS in India was co-ordinated by their office in New Delhi, headed by a field director who reported to the overseas director in London.

AIDPLUS (INDIA) had been talking about the possibility of raising funds in India for at least 15 years. The programme officers felt that if money were raised in India, there would be greater accountability and greater involvement of Indians in the work of AIDPLUS.

At an AIDPLUS management committee meeting held in Madras in December 1988, Mark Collet briefed the team about his plans to initiate a market research study. He said that the objective of the study was to provide quality information, which would be used to design a strategic plan to gradually Indianise AIDPLUS's resource base.

F.1.3   The Argument for Indian Fund-raising

The Indian voluntary sector is made up of thousands of societies and trusts of various religious and ideological persuasions. Despite the excellent work done by many of these agencies, the voluntary sector in India lacks credibility and is treated with suspicion by government agencies and the powerful Indian media. The main reason for this is the overwhelming dependence of most of these agencies on foreign aid, estimated to be in the region of Rs 50 billion (approximately £170,000,000) per year.

Due to this dependence, and complacency created by it, most NGOs have been content doing low profile work with foreign funding. Most foreign funding agencies are bound by commitments to their donor base, which has its own understanding of Third World development. This is despite the fact that many agencies like AIDPLUS spend considerable time and effort educating their donor constituencies.

Of far greater importance than the quantum of funds that could be raised in India, was the principle of moving towards self-reliance, which is the very basis of all development work.

The research team interviewed the top management of AIDPLUS (INDIA) and isolated the following motivations for wanting to start fund-raising in India. The strength of each motivation is indicated by the weighted score attached to it:

Rank	Motivation	Score
1	Getting the mandate of the Indian public for AIDPLUS's work in India	13
2	Create awareness about AIDPLUS's work in India	12
3	Create a corporate image for AIDPLUS in India	10
4	Autonomy through Indian money	9
5	Provide credibility for lobbying with government in India	5
6	International lobbying	2

It appeared from this study that the real reasons for wanting to start fund-raising in India were 'political' and 'moral' in nature rather than 'economic'.

AIDPLUS (INDIA) Society would act as a leader and catalyst in the field of local fund-raising. Utmost encouragement would be given to NGOs which wished to raise their own funds. Experience would be shared and capabilities strengthened.

AIDPLUS (INDIA) Society's thinking on fund-raising in India was based on a three-pronged strategy, which centred around awareness creation and involvement of the public in development issues, detailed as follows:

- **Charity giving** which meant raising funds from the public through media appeals, sponsored events, community link funding, payroll giving, schools, legacies, pledge giving and trusts, direct mail and a variety of innovative techniques such as credit cards, and mutual benefit marketing.
- **Charity products trading** which involved commercial activities requiring skills and endowments of project partners; trading of products and artifacts through a national network of shops; Design of exhibitions of rural arts and traditional art forms packaged for the urban market.
- **Inviting public participation** AIDPLUS aimed to provide a platform for concerned Indians to donate their time for, and to get an exposure to various development activities, as a means of involving the public in the work of AIDPLUS (INDIA). Some suggestion were organising alternative tourism packages such as summer camps for students in project areas; summer placement assignments for students of professional courses from centres of excellence; social sabbaticals for professionals who would be invited to donate professional time, underwritten by their companies.

F.2   MARKET RESEARCH FINDINGS

Mark Collet received a market research report from the Indian Market Intelligence Corporation (IMIC), one of India's leading research agencies. They had defined the Indian charity market in terms of the four metro cities (Delhi, Calcutta, Chennai, Mumbai) and five regional cities with populations of over 100,000.

Data had been collected using questionnaires, from individuals and corporations, and qualitative data had been collected using individual depth interviews and focus group discussions.

F.2.1   Attitudes to Charity in India

The Indian concept of charity has strong, religious overtones. However, it has been reduced to the ritual of feeding the poor on certain occasions or giving alms to wandering mendicants to invoke their blessings.

Collet felt that middle class Indians, who see poverty on a daily basis, would not be moved enough by the phenomenon to do something about it. That too, in a country where asceticism and poverty are sanctioned by religion. Knowing India as well as he did, Collet knew that there were ethnic and cultural barriers which would differentiate the fund-raising marketing campaign in India from similar campaigns in Europe and America.

F.2.1.1   *Western Assumptions*

Although, clearly, people in India gave money for charitable work, mainly for religious reasons as in Europe, it was apparent that there was a subtle cultural difference. To understand these cultural differences, Collet commissioned a separate study by INTERVENTION (INDIA) Pvt. Ltd., an agency which specialises in culturally-adapted social market research.

The director of this agency had pointed out that it would be fallacious to equate notions of Indian charity with notions of Western charity. The Western notion of charity came from pre-Christian, (Jewish, Greek and Roman) and Christian culture.

F.2.1.2   Hindu Notions of Charity

From expert interviews carried out by the agency, it was shown that the Hindu concept of **daan** (gift) differs considerably from the Western notion of charity. It is necessary to delink oneself from the item being given before it is handed over to a person worthy to receive it.

The Western concept of exchange tells us: 'When two parties enter into voluntary trade, both their utilities are increased'. The Hindu system obviously goes contrary to this idea; to fit the Hindu behaviour within a Western framework, we have to understand that the donor is 'purchasing' a 'spiritual good' in return for his gift.

One of the implications of this principle is that the donor has no right to question the manner in or the purpose to which his donation was applied.

Collet made a note to do some further probes to find out whether donors would value the right to know how their money was spent, because this was one of the important 'after-sales-service' items in the West.

The word *daan* (gift) is accompanied by two other words which probably complete the complex notion of Indian charity. These words are *yajna* (sacrifice) and *tapaha* (penance).

'Acts of sacrifice, charity and penance are not to be given up: they must be performed. Indeed, sacrifice, charity and penance purify even the great souls'.

How could AIDPLUS benefit from these insights which have a powerful influence on the way even modern Indians think?

We are told that 'When charity to the poor is given out of compassion, and the poor man is not worth giving charity to, then there is no spiritual advancement. . . . First you recognize the potential recipient's capabilities and then give him. . .that is *daan*'.

The IMIC's qualitative research showed that one of the 'counter-arguments' used by people approached for donations are that the poor misuse the donated money by drinking and gambling. AIDPLUS would have to use powerful communication to show that donors' money would be used for carefully planned activities under skilled supervision, and that there was no chance of misuse of the money.

Lok Kalyan Samiti and HelpAge, Delhi based NGOs supporting the elderly had been successfully using traditional Hindu ideas of reverence for elders, in their appeals.

The IMIC's research revealed that in India there is a notion of 'spiritual banking' and charitable giving is associated with:

★   help in times of need.
★   'It could happen to me (disasters)'.
★   'buying' protection.
★   providing safety from evil.

The more advanced concepts show:

★   a notion of 'opening an account with God', in which all charitable acts are 'credited'.
★   a belief that charitable giving guarantees a better life in the next birth.

The findings of the research showed some very down-to-earth and practical motivations for giving to charity in an economy that has functioned for years on the basis of the paradigm, 'REGULATION, ENFORCEMENT, and PUNISHMENT'.

In a command economy such as pertains in India, it is only natural that those who create wealth will seek loopholes to beat the system.

In this pursuit, charitable giving would be viewed as a means of getting income tax exemptions, and converting unaccounted or 'black money'. It was common for individuals to offer money to registered charities and ask for a receipt for three times the amount.

The findings of research also showed the development of a series of 'counter-arguments' against the general appeal for charitable giving.

* ★ 'They (recipients of monetary donations) can't be trusted. The money will probably be used for gambling and drinking.'
* ★ 'Funds never reach those for whom they are intended.'
* ★ 'I don't have enough to spare.'
* ★ 'There are many other demands on my earnings.'
* ★ 'My donation will be just a drop in the ocean.'

F.2.2   Preferred Causes and Issues

The focus group discussions conducted by IMIC indicated the following causes and issues (in order of preference) favoured for charitable support:

* Disasters.
* Helping the helpless and abandoned.
* Helping the physical handicapped.
* Poverty alleviation.
* Human capital—education and health.
* Rural development.
* Temple construction.

Important criteria for selection of causes or issues appeared to be the visibility of the need, and the conviction that urgent action is required.

Suggestions from focus group participants that in the case of disasters, photographs of the affected areas would convey a sense of the scale of damage, confirmed that visual communications can influence people to donate in response to disasters.

The gender issue which ranked first on AIDPLUS's list of priorities was viewed with mixed feelings by the various discussion groups.

Family 'disputes' (which subsume ill-treatment of women) were viewed strictly as family affairs, to be settled privately by the family. The notion of social action against the ill-treatment of women appeared to be alien, and appeared to be the sole preserve of traditional social mechanisms such as village elders' council and the panchayat.

F.2.3   Donating Behaviour Motivation

An analysis of the main reasons for making the most recent donation among 890 respondents showed that there were five major groups of motivations. These were:

- Emotional pull.
- Impulse.
- Rational.
- Compulsion (Peer pressure, what will others think?).
- Tradition (or habit, and the advice of elders).

Although a list of reasons with the proportion of respondents favouring them was given by the IMIC, the significance of these proportions had not been tested, and one needed to be careful about making inferences.

However, it was clear that religion dominated the whole area of charitable giving, although secular giving was indicated where the credibility of the organisation could be established beyond doubt.

There was a pervasive feeling that in religious giving, it is important to give without much rational justification. What happens to the donation is unimportant, even if it is suspected that the money is being used inefficiently. The attitude, however, was different when it came to secular giving. The public needed to have proof that their money was being used efficiently.

One of the challenges of a communication programme for AIDPLUS in India was to build a strong aura of credibility and integrity, as in the UK, so that people would give to AIDPLUS and not worry about the use of their money.

Although the evidence is not overwhelming, there are indications that Indians associate charitable giving with life-stage milestones such as births, weddings, deaths, and other auspicious functions.

F.2.4   Donation of Personal and Professional Time

The market research agency conducted a questionnaire survey in four metropolitan cities, using a stratified random sampling method.

As many as 49 per cent of the 452 respondents were willing to offer professional or technical services, and the proportion of 184 women at 55 per cent willing to offer such services was higher than 44 per cent of the 268 male respondents.

A majority (75 per cent) of the respondents said that they would donate their professional or technical services for the sake of satisfaction while a few expected to be compensated, at least for their expenses. Some (11 per cent) looked for positions of power in the voluntary organisations, while others (12 per cent) for glory—recognition, honour, award.

F.3   THE OBJECTIVES OF THE MARKETING PROGRAMME

Mark Collet turned to a fresh sheet on his scribbling pad. He decided to make a list of the objectives for starting up the marketing programme.

From the exercise on the motivations of the top management discussed earlier, it was clear to Collet, that the AIDPLUS (INDIA)'s marketing programme for fund-raising was not solely concerned with raising money. An equally important objective was to communicate with the people of India and get them involved in the work of AIDPLUS (INDIA).

The **purpose** of AIDPLUS (INDIA)'s fund-raising programme was to:

* **Reduce dependence on foreign money,** thus leading to the **goal** of
* **Sustainable development work.**

F.3.1   Reducing Dependence

The level of AIDPLUS (INDIA)'s funding, all of it from the UK, was Rs 5 crores (or Rs 50 million) in 1990, which at a conversion rate of Rs 50 to the £Stg, amounted to £Stg 1 million. There was no way that this huge amount could be substituted with locally raised Indian money overnight. It would not even be realistic to say that it could be done by the end of five years, because the amount required annually for programme expenditure was growing each year at an estimated 10 per cent.

Programme Expenditure	1990	1991	1992	1993	1994	1995
(Rupees in Millions)	50.0	55.0	60.0	67.0	73.0	81.0

However, Collet decided that it might be reasonable to say that a third of the amount required in 1995 could be raised locally if AIDPLUS (INDIA) got down to work fast. Even this amount would boost the confidence of AIDPLUS (INDIA)'s staff and this would be reflected in the kind of issues they selected for their work. They had to start somewhere.

He knew that initially AIDPLUS (INDIA) would have to invest in capacity building for fund-raising, a completely new activity. He contacted Anjali Menon, who was working for an advertising agency, and had shown interest in joining AIDPLUS (INDIA) as the fund-raising manager, even though it meant a 20 per cent cut in her salary.

F.3.2   Ways and Means

Collet, in consultation with Anjali Menon, decided that in the first year, AIDPLUS (INDIA) would be able to raise only 1 per cent of the total programme expenditure of Rs 50 million. He was aware that by 1995, he would have to build up the fund-raising revenue to a third (Rs 27 million) of the project programme expenditure of Rs 81 million. He would also have to commit himself to a fund-raising expenditure of Rs 4 million, which would give an acceptable expense ratio of about 7 per cent. This was another way of saying that it would cost one rupee to raise seven rupees, or Rs 15 to raise Rs 100.

AIDPLUS (INDIA) would concentrate on the first year's task of raising Rs 500,000, out of which Rs 400,000 would come from what appeared to be an easy source—the sale of greetings cards. Several other agencies—WWF (Worldwide Fund for Nature), CRY (Child Relief and You), HelpAge and UNICEF had been in the market for several years now. The remaining amount would come from direct mail. Collet knew that in Europe, 80 per cent of charity income came from direct mail.

Anjali Menon was sceptical about greetings cards. She was particularly doubtful about Collet's idea of using only Indian art card paper, which looked slightly shabby compared to foreign art cards. AIDPLUS (INDIA) did not want to support the use of imported paper. She pointed out that customers bought

Table F.1
AIDPLUS (INDIA) Income and Expenditure Estimates (1990–95)

Years	1990	1991	1992	1993	1994	1995
Programme Expenditure (Rupees in million)	50	55	60	67	73	81
Programme Expenditure percentage to raise	1%	3%	8%	14%	23%	33%
Income to be raised (Rupees in million)	0.5	1.65	4.8	9.38	16.79	27
Estimated Expenditure (Ruppes in million)	1.0	4.4	2.4	2.6	3.4	4
Est. Exp./income %	200	267	50	27.7	20.2	14.8
Inc.: Exp. ratio	0.5	0.38	2.0	3.6	4.9	6.8

greetings cards to satisfy their needs, not to support the high ideals of organisations like AIDPLUS (INDIA). She also reminded Collet that the sale of greetings cards required some experience in distribution channel management, which AIDPLUS (INDIA) did not have.

Anjali was equally sceptical about the direct mail plan. She felt that though this was a popular form of marketing in Europe and America, in India it was still a novelty, with very low response rates. However, she agreed to go ahead with the plan. The first year's risk was very low indeed with a target of raising only Rs 500,000.

F.4 IMPLEMENTATION

Anjali Menon joined AIDPLUS (INDIA) as the fund-raising manager, and had two British consultants from AIDPLUS (INTERNATIONAL) to help her set up her department. Anjali put two staff members on the job of collecting addresses of supporters of AIDPLUS (INDIA) from their archives. Within a month, they had assembled an impressive list of nearly 11,000 addresses.

She hired an executive to manage her database, and decided to work through a management consultancy firm in Bangalore called ALTERNATE MARKETING for greetings cards production and marketing.

F.4.1 Greetings Cards

The idea was to use Bangalore as a test market for greetings cards and proceed cautiously on the basis of the first year's experience. The costing of the greetings cards, prepared by ALTERNATE MARKETING was as follows:

Table F.2
Cost/Benefit Estimates of the Greetings Cards Venture

	No. of Cards	Sales Price/Card	Amount (in Rupees)
A : SALES			
Sales Planned	350,000	Rs 5.00	1,750,000
Sales Expected (80%)	280,000	Rs 5.00	1,400,000
B : COSTS		Cost/Card	
Cost of Production		Rs 2.00	700,000
Promotion and Advertising		0.30	105,000
Administration		0.64	224,000
Total		Rs 2.94	1,029,000
A-B: INCOME			371,000
Inventory carried over to next season	70,000		

If ALTERNATE MARKETING succeeded in selling 80 per cent of the year's production of 350,000 greetings cards at Rs 5 per card, and if the cost of production were kept below Rs 3, AIDPLUS (INDIA) would generate an income of over Rs 300,000 from this operation.

F.4.2   Direct Mail

The creative director of Anjali's former company offered the services of their copy writer and their layout artist, with whose help Mark Collet and Anjali finalised a design for a mailer.

They were careful to avoid the flashy suggestions of the layout artist, knowing that prospective supporters would get put off by very loud multi-coloured appeals on expensive paper.

The appeal was very simple. The copy read, 'Poverty has many faces. You can help to change the face of your city'. They were giving the supporters 'control' over what was happening around them, because research suggested that people were frustrated that they were no longer in control of the chaos that was happening in their very own environment.

Anjali offered potential supporters a 'shopping list' from which they could pick the level they could afford and send their contributions with a coupon giving their latest address and phone numbers. Those who couldn't send money were encouraged to send the addresses of five friends.

F.5   RESULTS OF THE CAMPAIGN

One year later, Mark Collet and Anjali Menon took stock of the results of their campaign.

F.5.1   The Greetings Cards Campaign: A Failure

It was unrealistic to have launched a greetings card campaign thinking that people would buy the card because of AIDPLUS (INDIA)'s international reputation. People never give money to organisations. They give money to causes, and when the fund-raising technique is something like greetings cards, the customer demands value for money. The paper on which AIDPLUS (INDIA)'s cards were printed looked shabby and customers were not interested. With great difficulty, 85,000 greetings cards were sold against a target of 2,80,000. Anjali realised that you have to establish a brand name before consumers can recognise it, and buy it.

F.5.2   Direct Mail: A Runaway Success

Their first mailing raised Rs 264,000 at an average rate of Rs 1,200 per donor. Direct mail was an opportunity to communicate with AIDPLUS (INDIA)'s supporters on a regular basis, and Anjali found that those who gave once were happy to give money again, provided they got information about how their money was spent. People wanted to feel that they were contributing in some small way to influencing the situation around them. AIDPLUS (INDIA) had become a vehicle for change, and it empowered people. If AIDPLUS (INDIA)'s campaigns had relied on guilt and pity, they would have never made a dent. In a country like India, with poverty all around, people were too insulated against it. But they were prepared to give money if it meant that it would make them feel good about it!

F.6   IMPORTANT LESSONS

Mark Collet's term as director had come to an end and he was writing up his handing-over notes. He included a special note on fund-raising and decided to put down on paper what he thought were the most important lessons he had learned.

F.6.1   Greetings Cards

There were three important segments to be taken into account in the sale of greetings cards. These were:

- The corporate market.
- The wholesale market.
- The retail market.

Companies were prepared to buy greetings cards in bulk, provided they were of high quality, as their corporate images were at stake. The fact that the money was going to a charity was not unimportant, but it was not the deciding factor. Collet had found that most companies expected the cards to be customised by having their logos and addresses printed inside. This was offered as a free service.

Each city had one or two centres which functioned as the wholesale market for greetings cards. Business was very brisk here and competition fierce. The wholesalers were interested only in established brands and expected heavy discounts from new entrants in the market. AIDPLUS (INDIA) had not reckoned on such a heavy initial cost to establish their brand.

The retail market had to be managed with a small sales force in each city, to ensure that the cards got displayed in a vantage point in the stores, and to ensure that sales were monitored and payments followed up after the agreed credit period.

F.6.2   Direct Mail

Building the initial database for cold-mailing was the most important task. Collet found that many young, upwardly mobile professionals quickly became dedicated supporters, as this gave them a feeling of being in control to some extent of the chaos surrounding them.

All copy and images were carefully monitored by Collet to ensure that the transaction was not a sale of victims or extreme poverty and deprivation. On the other hand, cheerful images gave the potential donor or sponsor a feeling that he or she was getting the opportunity to fulfill himself or herself.

Collet learned that retaining old supporters was an important aspect of supporter-base management, because it took considerable time and effort to recruit a new sponsor or donor. Supporters appreciated being able to visit projects and seeing for themselves what their support had achieved. Opportunities for such visits were built into the direct mail communications.

This case study should offer food for thought for NGOs engaged in fund-raising. There are a number of theoretical propositions which become apparent. A thorough investigation and understanding of what motivates different categories of donors to support charitable causes is an essential pre-condition of any fund-raising campaign. The resulting findings must be used to provide the base for careful target segmentation.

Part IV

A CASM Experimental Exercise

A CASM Strategy to Reduce the Incidence of Female Genital Mutilation

Hermione Lovel

The objective of this exercise is to encourage readers of this manual to attempt designing:

A CASM STRATEGY TO REDUCE THE INCIDENCE
OF FEMALE GENITAL MUTILATION (FGM)

We trust that working through this manual and in particular through the various case studies will make readers keen to experiment with designing a CASM strategy. We invite enterprising readers to try their skills in the context of what is a rather complex problem, namely female genital mutilation (FGM). FGM seriously harms the health of millions of women and their children.

We provide detailed background data of the various aspects of FGM in the hope that this social problem will engage the ingenuity of readers to produce an effective CASM campaign that will succeed in bringing about the decline and ultimately the elimination of FGM practices.

Please submit your CASM plan latest by 1 July 2000 to:

Dr Hermione Lovel
Department of General Practice
Rusholme Health Centre
Walmer Street
MANCHESTER M15 5NP

A committee of experts will examine the submissions and award three prizes:

1st prize : £Stg . 350
2nd prize : £Stg . 200
3rd prize : £Stg . 100

Awards will be announced by 1 December 2000.

EX.1   FGM AND ITS BACKGROUND

EX.1.1   The Negative Health Effects, How Many Girls and Women are Affected by it?[1]

At least 2 million girls per year are estimated to be at risk of genital mutilation adding to the 120 million girls and women who are estimated to have already undergone this procedure.[2]

EX.1.2   What is Female Genital Mutilation?

FGM is a deeply-rooted traditional practice. It is also a form of violence against girls and women that has serious physical, health and psycho-sexual health consequences.

Many women appear to be unaware of the relationship between FGM and its health consequences, in particular the complications affecting sexual intercourse and childbirth which occur many years after mutilation has taken place. Moreover, in many cases, women have been conditioned socially to accept the practice and the pain it causes. Although it does seem that some traditional practitioners are aware of the health problems of FGM, they perpetuate myths to make women believe that the problems are normal. In Sierre Leone, for example, traditional practioners know that the scar tissue will not usually yield for the first child and so have propagated the myth that it is usual to lose the first child at birth.

Female genital mutilation comprises all procedures that involve partial or total removal of the female external genitalia and/or injury to the female genital organs for cultural or any other non-therapeutic reasons.

EX.1.3   Female Genital Mutilation Practices

FGM encompasses a range of procedures including the excision of the prepuce (and fold of skin above the clitoris), the partial or total excision of the clitoris (clitoridectomy) and labia, and the stitching and narrowing of the vaginal orifice (infibulation). Excision of the clitoris or of the clitoris and labia minora is performed in approximately 80 per cent of girls and women who undergo genital mutilation. Infibulation—the most extreme form of mutilation—involves the complete removal of the clitoris and labia minora, together with the inner surface of the labia majora. The two sides of the vulva are then stitched together with thorns or silk or catgut sutures, so that when the skin of the remaining labia majora heals a bridge of scar tissue forms over the vagina and the clitoris. Sometimes the clitoris is cut off, which can lead to very severe bleeding of the clitoral artery. A small opening is preserved, by the insertion of a foreign body, to allow the passage of urine and menstrual blood. The legs are sometimes bound together for several weeks to allow the scar

---

[1]Derived from WHO/FREH/WHD/96.10.

[2]This figure has been rounded off from estimates derived from different sources including Tonbla N. (1995). *Female Genital Mutilation: A Call for Global Action*, New York and the Lexington Women International Network.

tissue to form. Since a physical barrier has been created, during sexual intercourse the infibulated woman has to undergo gradual dilation by her husband over a period of days, weeks or even months. This painful process does not always result in successful vaginal penetration and the opening may have to be re-cut. At childbirth, the woman has to be cut once more (defibulation) to allow the passage of the baby. After birth the raw edges may again be sutured (re-infibulation). Other mutilation procedures include introcision (the enlargement of the vaginal opening by tearing or cutting the perineum), the pricking, piercing, incising or cauterizing by burning of the clitoris and/or labia, and the scraping of surrounding tissue of the vaginal orifice (angurya cuts) or cutting off the anterior and sometimes posterior vaginal wall (gishiri cuts), and the insertion of salt in the vagina.

EX.1.4   When is FGM Done?

The age at which FGM is performed varies widely, depending on the ethnic group and geographical location. In some groups it is performed on babies; more commonly it is carried out when the girls are between the ages of 4 and 10 years but it may also be carried out in their adolescence or even at the time of marriage or during the first pregnancy. The operations, which often last about 15–20 minutes, are carried out with special knives, scissors, scalpels, pieces of glass or razor blades. The instruments may be re-used without cleaning. The operations are often performed by an elderly woman in the community, specially designated for this task or by traditional birth attendants, although the services of health personnel such as midwives and doctors may also be called upon. Anaesthetics and antiseptics are often not used, and pastes containing herbs, local porridge or ashes are frequently rubbed on the wounds to stop the bleeding. Even when health workers perform the operation, it is difficult to locally anaesthetise the area as numerous very painful injections need to be administered in an extremely sensitive area and local anaesthesia may still not be effective even after extensive administration. Unintended additional damage is often caused because of the use of crude tools, poor light, poor eyesight of the practitioner, and septic conditions, or because of the struggle put up by the girls and women during the procedure.

In Sudan, a woman may be 're-circumcised' after childbirth before returning to her husband. It is also said that in some areas, for example, in parts of Sudan, older women making themselves ready to go on pilgrimage to one of the holy cities often seek to be re-infibulated.

EX.1.5   What is the Geographical Distribution?

Most of the girls and women who have undergone mutilation live in 28 African countries. In one form or another it is practised by many ethnic groups from the East to the West coast of Africa, in the Southern parts of the Arabian peninsula, along the Persian Gulf, and increasingly found, due to migration, amongst the populations of Europe, Australia, Canada and the United States of America. It is also reported to be practised by Dandi Bohra Muslims who live in India and the UK and amongst Muslims in Malaysia and Indonesia. The severest form, infibulation, is widespread in Somalia, northern Sudan and Djibouti and has been reported in Ethiopia, Eritrea, northern Kenya and some parts of Mali and parts of northern Nigeria. 'Sealing' of the labia, performed sometimes in some groups in Gambia, has the same effect of causing the skin of the labia to join together permanently. Internal vaginal cuts (introcision) was documented amongst some aboriginal communities in Australia but is not considered to be current practice in this group.

Within a country the practice is often conducted only by particular ethnic groups. Within that ethnic group frequently 90–100 per cent of girls and women are affected. Recently questions on 'female circumcision' (FGM) have been incorporated into demographic health surveys, for example, in Sudan, Eritrea, Egypt, Mali[3] and so accurate prevalence data is gradually becoming available.

EX.1.6   Why is it Done?

It is not known when or where the tradition of female genital mutilation originated and a variety of reasons (socio-cultural, psycho-sexual, hygienic, aesthetic, and religious) are given for maintaining it. Female genital mutilation is practised by followers of a number of different religions, including Muslims and Christians (Catholics, Protestants and Copts), by Animists and also by non-believers in the countries concerned. The practice is deeply embedded in local traditional belief systems. It is important to note that neither the Bible nor the Koran prescribe the practice, although it is frequently carried out in some Muslim communities in the genuine belief that it forms part of Islam.

EX.1.7   Physical Consequences

Female genital mutilation frequently results in short- and long-term health consequences. The effects depend on the extent of cutting, the skill of the operator, the cleanliness of the tools, the environment, and the physical condition of the girl or woman concerned. Girls and women undergoing the more severe forms of mutilation are particularly likely to suffer serious and long-lasting complications.

Short-term complications include severe pain, injury to adjacent tissue, bleeding, shock, acute urine retention, fracture or dislocation (due to struggle), infection and failure to heal. Some girls die. In one part of West Africa it is said that mothers wait anxiously to see their daughters return from the initiation ceremony in the dancing procession, always fearing the worst; people talk of a sister or a friend who died during the circumcision ceremony.

Long-term complications include difficulty in passing urine, recurrent urinary tract infection, pelvic infection, infertility, keloid scar, abscesses and cysts, clitoral neuroma, difficulties in menstruation, callus formation in the vagina, fistulae (holes or tunnels) between the bladder and the vagina or the rectum and vagina, painful sexual intercourse, difficulty in sexual relations, difficulty with providing gynaecological care in remote areas, problems in pregnancy and childbirth because of the tough scar tissue and delay in childbirth leading to stillbirth or possibly maternal death.

EX.1.8   Sexual and Mental Health Consequences

FGM can have a lifetime effect on the minds of those who have experienced it. There is little systematic information available. Current information is based on field observations and preliminary pilot studies.

---

[3]Except for Sudan there are no reliable revelence data on FGM.

Sexual relations may lead to bleeding from stretched scar tissue, new tears, and severe pain from damaged nerve tissue, orgasm may be lost. Despite such difficulties, women experience sexual desire and some degree of sexual enjoyment may be possible.

Prior to the mutilation girls may often be deceived, intimidated, coerced and suffer violence at the hand of trusted parents (often the mother) or other relatives (often aunts). In some instances they are forced to watch the mutilation of other girls. It is thus a major experience of fear, submission, inhibition and suppression of feelings and thinking. It becomes a vivid landmark in their mental development, the memory of which persists throughout life. Older women have said 'nothing since then has come close to the pain of that time'. Some have difficulty recalling and describing it but their tension and tears reflect the magnitude of emotional pain they silently endure at all times. Even with the family support they receive at the time, girls may feel anger, bitterness and betrayal at having been subjected to such pain. The loss of confidence and trust in family and friends may affect child-parent relationships and has implications for future intimate relationships with adults and with their own children. For many girls and women it is said the mental experience of genital mutilation and its aftermath are very similar to those following rape.

The experience of genital mutilation may be commonly associated with psychosomatic and mental problems, symptoms and disorders which affect a wide range of brain functions. Girls have reported disturbances in eating, sleep, mood and cognition. These were manifested in sleeplessness, nightmares, loss of appetite, weight loss or excessive gain, post-traumatic stress, panic attacks, mood instability and difficulties in concentration and learning. As they grow older, women may develop feelings of incompleteness, they may suffer from loss of self-esteem, depression, chronic anxiety, phobia, panic or even psychotic disorders. These may be compounded by the development of the serious long-term physical health effects of mutilation. Many women traumatized by their experience of genital mutilation have no acceptable means of expressing their fears and pains and suffer in silence.

THE POSITIVE SOCIAL DIMENSIONS OF THIS HARMFUL TRADITIONAL PRACTICE

Gold necklaces, gold bracelets, party dresses and many other new clothes, large amounts of cash and huge esteem all come to the girl who has just had FGM in areas where the girls are circumcised between 6 and 14 years of age and the ceremony is done in groups.

In Gambia, along all the little paths of the village and down the main road of the town, at the gateway of each house with a child of the right age, a flag flutters high on a flagpole to show how many girls are in the current ceremony.

Initiation to membership of the key women's societies is an important feature of the FGM ceremony and ritual in West Africa. Only when they have been through it do girls truly 'belong' and their mothers can become senior members of these societies. In such area 300 or more girls are involved at any one time. It is a great honour if a famous 'circumciser' visits from a neighbouring area or country to perform the cutting.

In some areas, young girls are taken away from villages into the remote rural areas for the ceremony. They are kept there for some weeks not just to heal but also to be taught about the duty of women to keep themselves clean and beautiful, how to keep their skin soft, their bodies supple, and their future husbands sexually satisfied. They may learn about looking after a home too. (In the past, some girls in Gambia were married within weeks of the ceremony. These days this is not often the case as girls are circumcised at a much younger age and they now marry when they are older).

'Traditional sex education' as this procedure could be termed has been documented in a number of areas independent of FGM. In Uganda (Entebbe) it was found to be an important role for the maternal aunt. Her job is first to prevent her niece from getting pregnant before marriage (with advice on traditional contraception, particularly using waist ties prepared in a special way and sworn to be effective). Her second job is to ensure pregnancy straight after marriage. There are stories of aunts lying under the marital bed to encourage the couple. This longstanding form of opportunity for young people to learn about sexual matters could easily be extended to HIV/AIDS prevention education and the health benefits of spacing births.

Girls of course feel grown-up after the ceremony. Often they live in areas where boys are circumcised at a similar pre-puberty/early puberty stage with similar flags and similar gifts. In many areas secrecy surrounds the rituals, participants are sworn to silence so there can never be any discussion of what has happened. For re-circumcision in the postpartum period, 'the scraping clean' of the vulva, there is the opportunity for a formal ritual to recognise a cleansing after the messy business of childbirth. In the religious domain of re-infibulation prior to visiting a holy city there is also the sense of making oneself clean before going to a place of God.

For the families of the girls it is seen as essential that the girls are circumcised before arrangements can be made for their marriage. In some groups, there is said to be no possibility of finding a husband for an uncircumcised daughter. However, in almost every group there seem to be a few girls who were never done (this is illustrated by the following sayings: 'I was too sickly as a baby/child'; 'I was done but not my sister'; 'Only three of the five girls were done').

In the societies where baby girls have their clitoris removed at 8 days of age (e.g., Ethiopia) this may be done on an individual basis without much ceremony, not in groups and certainly without any social education of the baby.

In many countries, it is said that the age of female genital mutilation is lowering, removing the positive aspect of sex and social education. In addition, in some areas, for example in parts of Egypt, the cutting is being medicalised, removing the 'group initiation' and often also causing more physical damage. The entire community may be involved in the public recognition of a daughter becoming grown-up by being asked to contribute presents and cash. Everyone knows it is a very expensive time for the parents.

EX.3   THE INTERESTED PARTIES

EX.3.1   The Traditional Excisors

Many of the traditional excisors in West Africa rely on the large group ceremonies for their income in the wet season when crops have been recently planted and not yet ready to be harvested. Ceremonies are planned some weeks in advance. The excisors are paid in cash (a moderate sum) but more importantly they also receive gifts (chickens etc.) and all the food, buckets, bowls and clothes sent generously with the girls but not needed during the days or weeks of the ceremony. It is this receipt of these goods which is so valuable to the excisors. These can be sold a few at a time, when prices are high during the rainy season and periods of food shortages.

In some areas many of the traditional excisors are also traditional birth attendants who deliver most babies locally. They have an interest in making sure that babies are safely delivered and so in some areas (e.g.,

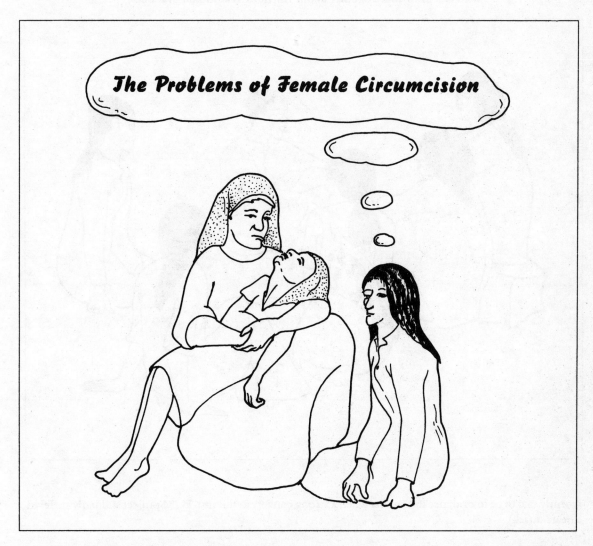

in part of Gambia) it is FGM awareness among the TBAs that has been the starting point of a programme to try to prevent FGM in the long-term. However, the few TBAs interviewed so far say that there are so many reasons for a delivery to go wrong that scarring from clitoral excision cannot be pointed out as the only reason.

The traditional excisors are very powerful ·not just as ascribed by others, but in their manner, bearing and personality. Their skill has been passed down the maternal line—from mothers to daughters. In parts of West Africa, if ever they decide to stop excising they must perform a special ceremony with the secret society. If they stop excising but do not perform the ceremony, it is believed that they will die (as was

Who Needs to Talk Together about Harmful Traditional Practices?

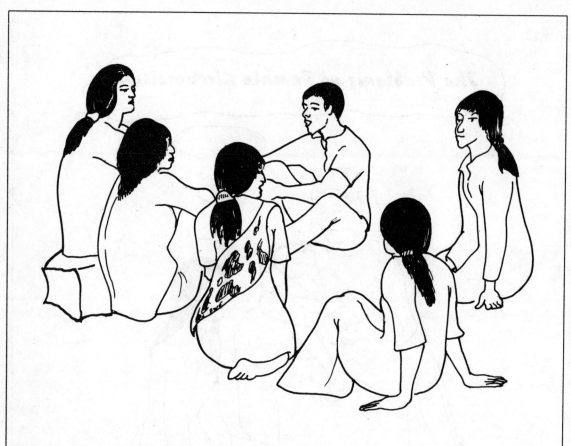

recently said to be in evidence in Gambia when a strong convert to the anti-FGM project suddenly suffered a heart-attack).

EX.3.2   The New Excisors

Increasingly trained health workers in countries where FGM is not yet illegal, and sometimes also when it is, are working as excisors. They claim to follow hygienic procedures, the ability to stop bleeding (which is not true as the clitoral artery is particularly difficult to suture) and charge a large fee. They rarely mention pain relief as they cannot do this either. As described above, it is very difficult to anaesthetise the clitoris under a local anaesthetic due to the extensive nerve supply and the need to apply multiple painful applications of the needle.

The New Role of the TBA

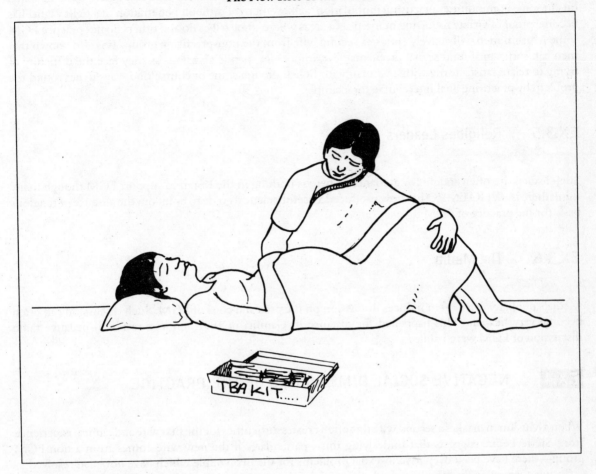

EX.3.3   The Mothers

Mothers often have a vested interest in getting their daughters 'done'. They want to avoid the fear 'the clitoris could grow into a male organ', or 'be cumbersome' to the hard agricultural work needed by an adult woman. They want their daughters to be marriageable. In secret society areas, mothers know that they will never hold a senior appointment until their daughters have been through the ceremony.

EX.3.4   The Men

Men clearly have an interest in marrying circumcised women; their mothers are said to tell them to marry only 'a clean circumcised' girl. It is said, however, that there are men who have been so disturbed by hearing the screams of their sisters 'being done' that they strongly refuse to allow their daughters to be operated on. In some communities practising infibulation, achievement of difficult penetration of a tight vagina has become proof of virility following marriage. In areas where some tribes do and others do not practice FGM some Muslim men will actively choose a second wife from the non-practising group. It is also known that men can suffer profound sexual problems, fear, impotence, penile abrasions as they face the difficulty of trying to relate satisfactorily with a woman with FGM, though some of course find ways to get round the problem by practising anal intercourse for example.

EX.3.5   Religious Leaders

Such leaders are often sought for guidance. There is nothing in the Koran to support FGM though many think there is. WHO EMRO has now produced a useful practical guide to point out the absence of religious basis for the practice of FGM.

EX.3.6   The Media

Media's publicity drive often induces discussion on the pros and cons of FGM. Such discussion can often become very heated. This happened for instance in Gambia in 1997 and as a result all negative radio discussion of FGM were banned.

EX.4   NEGATIVE SOCIAL DIMENSIONS OF THE PRACTICE

When a Muslim man takes a second wife this often creates difficulties for the first wife and clinical experience from Sierre Leone suggests that underlying this—particularly if the new wife comes from a non FGM group—there have been deep psychosexual problems for the first couple which have not been resolved.

To what extent such difficulties lead to a promiscuity of extra-marital relations, to STD transmission, including HIV/AIDS is not known.

Studies have suggested that FGM does not reduce pre-marital sex and there is discussion whether it could even increase it.

EX.5   SOME APPROACHES THAT ARE TAKING PLACE IN SOME AREAS

In some areas it is said infibulation is reducing and instead clitoridectomy is being done. However, although this might be termed more minor it can, in fact, be worse. Cutting the clitoral artery can cause life threatening bleeding which is difficult to stop. In infibulation, the clitoris may often simply be tucked inside, maybe leaving residual sensation as well. There is one anecdotal report from Surinam in South America that FGM has been replaced by a ritual using a peanut. In Gambia one FGM project is attempting to restructure puberty rites into 'initiation without mutilation'. Another approach is through generating alternative income for the excisors. This is also being tried in Gambia.

In some countries, a legal approach has been taken. Child Protection has been invoked in UK (to prevent young girls from being taken abroad expressly for FGM) via the Children Act. In Egypt, health workers were legally prevented from undertaking FGM. This was then overturned and now is being taken to a Higher Court. At the local level one project is providing support (and moral support and protection) to about 50 families with a girl child deemed at risk.

Community education often in the context of women's health is the other approach, through youth groups, women's groups and for men. Religious leaders have also been brought together to discuss FGM in workshops and also local chiefs so they can support what is happening to prevent FGM and speak out when necessary. Only a few years ago FGM could never be spoken of in public so some steps forward have been taken.

WHAT OTHER METHODS CAN BE DESIGNED TO DISCOURAGE THE PRACTICE OF FGM? PLEASE LET US HAVE YOUR IDEAS ON THE SUBJECT!

EX.6   RECOMMENDED READING

Adebajo CO (1992). 'Female circumcision and other dangerous practices to women's health', M.N. Kisekka, *Women's Health Issues in Nigeria*, p. 17, Zaria, Tamaza Publishing Co.

El Dareer A. (1980). 'An epidemiological study of female circumcision in the Sudan' Thesis Department of Community Medicine, Faculty of Medicine, University of Khartoum, MS.

Department of Statistics (1979). *Sudan Fertility Survey*, Ministry of Economic and National Planning, Khartoum.

Department of Statistics (1989/1990). *Sudan Demographic and Health Survey*, Ministry of Economic and National Planning, Khartoum.

Opio A. (1986). 'Family planning practices traditional and modern in Uganda' (unpublished MSc dissertation), Institute of Child Health, University of London.

Toubia N. (1995). *Female genital mutilation: a call for global action*, New York, Rainbo.

WHO (1996). *Female Genital Mutilation*. Report of a WHO technical working group 17–19 July 1995. WHO/FRH/WHD/96.10.

Appendix

Reader's Questionnaire

Dear Reader,

We trust you find our manual interesting and are keen to know whether it helps you in your developmental activities.

We take the unconventional step to include a questionnaire in the hope that you will agree to complete and return it to the publishers. This will help us to ensure that future editions of this manual will be truly user-friendly and include exactly the items that interest our readers; moreover, we intend to establish a CASM network and possibly a CASM newsletter, if we find a demand for it.

Have you ever used CASM?   Yes   No?

If (yes) has it helped to reach your objectives?   Yes   No?

Do you work for a developmental agency?

(please give details)   NGO...

                                    GOVERNMENT DEPT?.......................

                                    INTERNATIONAL ORG?....................

Which of the section in this manual interested you most? ....

Which of the section in this manual interested you least? ....

Would you like to receive a CASM newsletter?   Yes   No

Would you like to attend a CASM training workshop?   Yes   No

What CASM issues would you like to have set out in greater detail?

....

....

....

Any other comments...

....

....

If you would like to join a CASM network and to exchange relevant experiences please indicate your

Name...

Address..

....

THANK YOU FOR DEVOTING YOUR TIME AND EFFORT
TO COMPLETE THIS QUESTIONNAIRE

Notes on Contributors

T. SCARLETT EPSTEIN has spent over 30 years studying and consulting Third World Development. She is a professional development economist and an experienced development anthropologist. Her publications include the classics: *Economic Development and Social Change in S. India; South India: Yesterday, Today and Tomorrow; Capitalism, Primitive and Modern, The Feasibility of Fertility Planning* and *Women, Work and Family* besides many articles in various journals. She has conducted numerous consultancies for international organisations, such as UNICEF, UNFPA, ILO, SAREC, NORAD, DANIDA as well as many NGOs. Since retiring from her Research Professorship at the University of Sussex, England, some years ago, she has acted as director of SESAC (Scarlett Epstein Social Assessment Consultancy), England, INTERVENTION (a management consulting agency with a focus on development), S. India and SOMRA (a social and market research agency), Bangladesh. Dr Epstein has pioneered the cultural-adaptation of social market research and social marketing and has published *The Manual for Culturally-Adapted Development Market Research in the Development Process* and *The Training Manual for Development Market Research Investigators*. She now specialises in conducting CASOMAR and CASM workshops for Third World trainers of indigenous personnel.

MARIE-THERESE FEUERSTEIN is a Senior Freelance Consultant in international health, primary health care, adult education and community development, with experience in reproductive health, human resource development, health systems development in South and Central America, Africa, South East Asia and the Asian and Pacific regions. Originally trained as a nurse/midwife, with degrees and fieldwork in health, community development and adult education, she is now a Senior Consultant to WHO, UNDP, FAO, World Bank, and international NGOs. She is the author of the books *Partners in Evaluation, Turning the Tide, Safe Motherhood*, a district action manual, and *Poverty and Health* and numerous papers on health evaluation and community issues.

MITHILESHWAR JHA is Professor of Marketing at the Indian Institute of Management, Bangalore, India. He has a B.Tech. in Agricultural Engineering from G.B. Pant University, Pantnagar, India and has done his postgraduation and doctorate in Management at the Indian Institute of Management, Ahmedabad. He has about 18 years of teaching and industrial experience. He has published papers in Indian journals and has about a dozen cases to his credit. He has acted as consultant for international organisations like NORAD, Swiss Agency for Development Cooperation, Dhaka, Bangladesh and numerous leading Indian organisations. He has also conducted workshops and now specialises in conducting postgraduate level courses on social marketing.

HERMIONE LOVEL is Senior Lecturer in the Department of General Practice, a WHO collaborating Centre for Primary Health Care, at the University of Manchester, UK. She has set up and is Course Director of the MSc programme in Primary Health Care at the University of Manchester. She has qualifications and fieldwork experience in reproductive health, health services research, and customs and practices affecting health in sub-Saharan Africa, South Asia, North East Brazil, and parts of the eastern Mediterranean region.

Originally trained in biological sciences, social sciences, education, and public health, she has worked at the London School of Hygiene and Tropical Medicine (a collaborative programme with the Commonwealth Secretariat and Ghana); at the Institute of Development Studies, University of Sussex, in collaboration with SIDA/SAREC Sweden and the University of Ghana on a multidisciplinary health services research project in Ghana and later with the Ministry of Health in Ghana on a new National Primary Health Care Strategy; at the Centre for International Child Health, Institute of Child Health, London, where for 15 years she taught and then became course director of the Master's course in Mother and Child Health. Her current research work includes studies of reproductive morbidity in Sudan, (with WHO) developing protocols to identify and ameliorate the obstetric and psychosexual sequelae of FGM, finding out about the health needs of Somali refugees in the UK, and pregnancy health and its effect on the health of newborn babies in Zaire and Sri Lanka.

She has co-authored a number of books on district health care in developing countries including *My Name is To-day* (an illustrated discussion of child health, society, and poverty in less developed countries); *District Health Care*, which provides guidelines for planning, organisation and evaluation; and *Training material for Maternal and Child Health including Family Planning*. She has written numerous research papers on topics related to reproductive health.

AJIT MANI is managing director of INTERVENTION (India) Pvt. Ltd., a management consulting firm dedicated to the development sector. Before setting up INTERVENTION in 1992, he worked as director, social marketing in Sista's Pvt. Ltd., a mainstream advertising agency, as field director for South India, with ACTIONAID, a British charity, and with PRADAN (Professional Assistance for Development Action) and as action consultant to MYRADA in Karnataka. Ajit Mani is an alumnus of the Indian Institute of Management and Madras Christian College.

PATRICIO MORA is a Doctor of Medicine and Surgery from Cuenca State University, Ecuador, South America. After his graduation in 1983 he worked for two years as resident physician, intensive care unit, regional hospital, Cuenca before proceeding to work for three years as a vocational rehabilitation counsellor for the disabled with the Rehabilitation Services Commission, Toledo, Ohio, USA. Subsequently he worked as medical consultant in Peru and implemented a programme for tuberculosis control among the indigenous population and as vocational rehabilitation coordinator for the Louis Armstrong Rehabilitation Center, New York, USA until he became the health co-ordinator for PLAN INTERNATIONAL/UNFPA, Ecuador, responsible for the implementation of rural primary health projects.

ANNE OWITI is a trained nurse/midwife and as such ran a private clinic in Nairobi. In the course of her work she encountered the many serious problems that result from the spread of HIV\AIDS\STDs. As a result, she pioneered with the support from ACTION AID a novel Community Self-help Programme in Kibera, a large slum area in Nairobi. Her imaginative and multi-pronged approach has attracted not only attention within Kenya but also on the international scene.

SUSAN THOMAS has a postgraduate degree from TISS (Tata Institute of Social Sciences) and worked with Quantum Marketing, a leader in qualitative market research in India before joining INTERVENTION as a social research specialist.

About the Editor

T. SCARLETT EPSTEIN is currently a Director of three organisations—SESAC (Scarlett Epstein Social Assessment Consultancy), Hove, UK; INTERVENTION (Policy Consultants) Pvt. Ltd., Bangalore, India; and Somra Ltd., Dhaka, Bangladesh. She has previously been research Professor at the University of Sussex and a Visiting Professor at the universities of Minnesota and California and the Ben Gurion University of the Negev, Israel. In addition, Professor Epstein has served as a consultant to numerous national and international organisations including the World Bank, the OECD, UNICEF, FAO, ESCAP and the EU.

Dr Epstein has published a number of books including *Economic Development and Social Change in South India* (1962); *South India: Yesterday, Today and Tomorrow* (1973); *Women, Work and Family* (1986); *Improving NGO Development Programs* (1995); and *Village Voices: Forty Years of Rural Transformation in South India (1998)*. She has published more than fifty articles besides being the editor of a series entitled *Women in Development*, and of the *Newsletter for Small Rural Enterprises in Africa*, and *Rural Development in Practice*.